Contents

A guide to infectious diseases

M G BROOK

Senior Registrar, Department of Infectious and
Tropical Diseases, Royal Free Hospital, London

AND

M F McGHEE

General Practitioner, Castle Donington

RADCLIFFE MEDICAL PRESS
OXFORD

1870905601

© 1991 Radcliffe Medical Press Ltd
15 Kings Meadow, Ferry Hinksey Road, Oxford OX2 0DP

British Library Cataloguing in Publication Data

Brook, M. G.
A guide to infectious diseases
1. Communicable disease
I. Title   II. McGhee, M. F. (Michael Francis)
616.9
ISBN 1 870905 60 1

Typeset by Advance Typesetting Ltd, Oxford
Printed and bound in Great Britain

Preface

TEN years ago many doctors would have predicted the demise of
infectious diseases as an important specialty. Newer and more powerful
antimicrobial agents were providing the basis for an optimistic view that
all important infections would, sooner or later, be treatable. The appearance of novel infectious agents, such as the human immunodeficiency
virus (HIV), and the ability of some bacteria to acquire rapidly antibiotic
resistance have served to emphasize that however medical technology
improves, the pathogens will still be able to mutate and become resistant
to drugs. Many of the infections documented for years are still causing
disease and rising rates of foreign travel in the population (more than
250 million people travel worldwide annually) mean that the doctor
increasingly has to consider tropical infections in the differential
diagnosis of fever. Infectious diseases account for a fifth of morbidity in
primary care. Consultations due to infections and parasitic diseases
have increased by 25% in the last 10 years.

This book is not intended to be a comprehensive description of all
infectious disease, but rather a concise *aide-memoire* suitable as a rapid
reference on the more common and important illnesses. There are also
brief sections on epidemiology, public health and immunization which
should provide much of the information required by non-specialist
hospital doctors, medical students and general practitioners (GPs) alike.

MG Brook
MF McGhee
May 1991

CHAPTER 1

Epidemiology and public health aspects of infection

WHILST the diagnosis and management of infectious diseases may well be intellectually satisfying, the more mundane tasks associated with the prevention of such diseases are of equal or greater importance.

Modes of transmission of infection

Person-to-person spread

Droplet spread

Many infectious agents are present in high concentrations in respiratory secretions and are spread when a cough or sneeze releases aerosolized droplets into the atmosphere. These can then be inhaled by susceptible individuals. Anyone within 3 m (10 feet) or more of the index case is therefore at risk of a wide range of infections, including the childhood exanthematous illnesses, leprosy and streptococcal disease.

Faeco-oral transmission

Faeco-oral transmission is also a common means by which some infections are disseminated. It is a particularly important mode in children, people working in institutions or living in conditions of poor sanitation. The infectious agents, many of which do not cause diarrhoea, are secreted into the gut and taken up by the faeces. Failure to wash the hands after defaecation leads to contamination with organisms that may have a very low infectious dose. These can be transferred to others by direct hand-to-hand contact, and by contamination of the environment, particularly food. Such infections can also be transmitted when human sewage is allowed to contaminate food or water supplies. *Shigella* can cause infection when as few as 10 organisms are ingested. Other notable examples include hepatitis A virus and enteroviruses (which can also be spread by droplets). Many helminthic infections, such as hookworm and *Strongyloides*, are transmitted via faecally contaminated soil in the tropics.

Contamination of the environment

Contamination of the environment can be particularly problematic within hospitals where ill patients are at risk of being infected with dangerous pathogens shed by infected individuals. In many cases, the situation is not recognized until several people have been infected. *Streptococcus pyogenes* may be harboured harmlessly on the skin or in the upper airways of a patient or health care attendant. Spread to the environment may eventually lead, often via others acting as intermediary carriers, to infection of a third party manifest as erysipelas, cellulitis, tonsillitis and a variety of other diseases. Staphylococci (including the methicillin-resistant variety) and Gram-negative organisms are also routinely transmitted in this way. Large outbreaks of streptococcal skin sepsis have been recognized in army recruits who were infected by contaminated gymnasium equipment.

Food-borne transmission

Whilst the majority of infections transmitted by food contamination are of the faeco-oral or animal-derived type, some infectious agents can be spread from person to person by food contaminated in other ways, for instance, respiratory secretions contaminating food can lead to staphylococcal food poisoning or streptococcal tonsillitis.

Contamination with body fluids and tissues

The most obvious example of contamination by body fluids and tissues is sexually transmitted diseases (STDs). Other avoidable examples include sharps injury, the contamination of wounds and eczematous skin by a patient's blood, urine, faeces or saliva, the transfusion of infected blood and blood products, organ and tissue donation and the use of incompletely sterilized re-usable instruments. In this way, the human immunodeficiency virus (HIV), hepatitis B virus and several other serious infections have been transmitted.

Close personal contact

In situations of close personal contact, the organism is transferred directly, usually from skin to skin, from source to new host. Head and body lice are routinely transmitted this way, and staphylococci can easily spread to wounds from a surgeon afflicted with a skin infection.

Zoonoses

Direct contact with an infected animal can be particularly dangerous when rabies is involved. *Coxiella burnetii* (Q fever), brucellosis, orf and cat-scratch disease are other examples.

Animals can also infect man via an arthropod vector. Lyme disease is acquired from deer and other animals by the intermediary tick. The tick can also spread encephalitis viruses (not in the UK) and *Coxiella burnetii*. Sandflies transmitting the agents of leishmaniasis is one of the many other cases where this route is important.

Strategies for the prevention of disease

There are several ways in which it is possible to improve the chances of individuals within the community avoiding illness as the result of contracting an infectious disease.

Immunization

Immunization is an important strategy in the prevention of infectious diseases, and it is dealt with in Chapter 17.

Personal fitness and health

High standards in nutrition, physical fitness and personal cleanliness have also had a large part to play in reducing the incidence of diseases, such as tuberculosis (TB), that were once common in the United Kingdom (UK). Cholera and typhoid are no longer endemic in the UK because of the excellent sewage and water supply system.

Isolation

The isolation of people suffering from the more severe transmissible diseases, such as diphtheria and meningococcal disease, can be arranged. In some less dangerous diseases, this can be achieved at home, but hospital isolation is required for many. However, merely putting a patient in a side room off a general ward will not necessarily contain the spread of chickenpox. Similarly, hand washing and other appropriate strategies are unlikely to contain methicillin resistant staph. aureus (MRSA) unless strictly implemented; indeed, many large hospitals have found this to their cost.

The containment of infection within the hospital calls for clear guidelines to cover all possibilities, and this should be confirmed by an infection control team. This body would normally consist of a microbiologist, senior specialist nurse and an infectious diseases specialist, if available. Isolation should be offered for all conditions known easily to be transmittable from person to person without a food or arthropod vector and particularly those associated with a high morbidity or mortality. The isolation ward should be in a specialist unit away from non-infected patients and staffed by experienced personnel. The room ventilation characteristics should ideally ensure air outflow to the atmosphere away from ward areas, and the room should be cleaned daily to prevent the accumulation of pathogens on the floor and work surfaces. Staff should wear protective clothing, including masks if necessary, at a level adequate for the degree of infectivity of the pathogen. Hands should be washed each time a staff member leaves the room, and body fluids and excreta disposed of in a safe manner.

Outbreaks of infection within the hospital (nosocomial disease) should be dealt with firmly by the infection control team who should have the power to dictate admissions and bed use during the period of control.

Education of all members of staff in the safe practices required to prevent cross-infection and about personal risk should be an integral part of hospital policy.

Control of infection in the community

Control of infection in the community is within the remit of the consultant in communicable diseases control (CCDC) [formerly medical officer for environmental health (Infection)]. All infections on the list of notifiable diseases (*see* Appendix 1) should, as a statutory requirement, be notified in writing via the local Environmental Health Office. These are then added to the national statistics correlated by the Office of Population Censuses and Surveys. Certain infections should be notified to the CCDC by telephone and these include suspected cases of meningococcal disease, diphtheria, Lassa fever and other notifiable viral haemorrhagic fevers, typhoid, cholera and open pulmonary tuberculosis. Effective early action can then be taken to prevent secondary cases and detect disease in the early incubating stages.

Epidemic control

When outbreaks cross geographical boundaries or are extensive, national bodies such as that at the Communicable Diseases Surveillance Centre exist to correlate information and intervene as necessary.

CHAPTER 2

Central nervous system infections

THE presence of central nervous system (CNS) signs, especially depressed consciousness, headache and confusion in the febrile patient, is a worrying clinical problem. The diagnosis can be relatively easy, as for example in the patient who has a generalized purpuric rash and board-like neck stiffness, signifying meningococcal disease. In the very young and elderly, the diagnosis is less obvious, as CNS infections can be extremely subtle in their presentation. In such cases, the doctor's threshold for active investigation should be very much lower. Additionally, systemic effects of infections, such as pneumonia or pyelonephritis, can also be associated with features suggestive of CNS infection.

The most common type of CNS infection is viral meningitis, a proportion of cases of which can be managed in the home providing the patient is frequently visited. However, when bacterial meningitis is suspected, the patient should be admitted to hospital as an emergency. Pre-admission administration of intramuscular (im) penicillin can make the difference between survival and death in meningococcal infection, when its potential benefit far outweighs any theoretical disadvantage.

Cerebral abscess

Causative agents

- *Streptococcus milleri* (60–70%).
- *Bacteroides* spp. (20–40%).
- Enterobacteriaceae (up to 30%).
- Fungi (up to 15%).
- *Staphylococcus aureus* (10–15%).
- Often polymicrobial.
- Tuberculomas related to infection with *Mycobacterium tuberculosis* are a rare cause.

Epidemiology and pathophysiology

- The majority of cases arise spontaneously, but a variable number (20–60%) has been reported secondary to infection in the ear, sinuses, and lungs (bronchiectasis).

Incubation period

● Unknown.

Clinical features

● The majority of patients present with symptoms and signs of a space-occupying lesion: headache, depressed consciousness and developing focal neurological signs.
● Fever is present in only 50%.
● Additional features include: meningism, evidence of raised intracranial pressure, and seizures in a minority.

Differential diagnosis

● Meningitis.
● Encephalitis.
● Cerebral toxoplasmosis.
● Cerebral malignancies.
● Head injury.
● Cerebrovascular accident (CVA).

Diagnosis

● The organism may be found in blood cultures, although many patients require craniotomy and drainage, in which case the agent will be identified by culture of aspirated pus.
● If this diagnosis is at all likely, the patient should be transferred to a centre with computerized tomography (CT) facilities.

Treatment

● Some abscesses resolve with medical therapy alone, using benzyl-penicillin (30–40 mg/kg, 4–6 hourly) usually with chloramphenicol (12–15 mg/kg, 6 hourly) and metronidazole (7.5 mg/kg, 8 hourly) intravenously (iv). This therapy may require change in the presence of a staphylococcal or fungal aetiology.
● Craniotomy and aspiration of the abscess cavity is carried out in most neurosurgical units.

Prevention

● Nil.

Acute bacterial meningitis

Causative agents

- *Haemophilus influenzae* under 5 years old.
- *Streptococcus pneumoniae*, *Neisseria meningitidis* and *Listeria monocytogenes* at any age.
- Group B streptococci and *Escherichia coli* in neonates.

Epidemiology

- *H. influenzae*, *N. meningitidis* and *S. pneumoniae* are droplet spread from asymptomatic carriers. These 3 agents account for the majority of the 2600 cases seen each year in the UK.
- *L. monocytogenes* can be acquired from food, particularly soft cheeses, chicken and pre-packed salads. This organism most commonly affects the young, elderly and immunocompromised.
- *S. pneumoniae* commonly occurs in patients with skull fractures and cerebrospinal fluid (CSF) leaks.
- *N. meningitidis* Group B occurs sporadically with small outbreaks. Groups A, C and W can produce epidemics but these are less common in developed countries. Children and young adults are most frequently affected. Winter peaks occur, and approximately 1000–1200 cases are seen each year in the UK.

Incubation period

- The incubation period varies among the organisms, but is usually 4–14 days.

Clincal features

- In those over the age of 1 year, symptoms include headache, fever up to 40°C, nausea/vomiting, photophobia and drowsiness, profound neck stiffness, and a positive Kernig's sign will usually be found.
- In children under 1 year of age, the signs can be much more subtle, in particular there may be no neck stiffness, although the fontanelles may be bulging.
- Meningitis caused by *H. influenzae* and *N. meningitidis* may be preceded by upper respiratory symptoms, and both, especially *N. meningitidis*, can be associated with purpuric rash.
- *N. meningitidis* can cause fulminating septicaemia, proceeding rapidly to death, again associated initially with a purpuric and, later, an echymotic eruption. Meningitis may not occur in such cases.

Differential diagnosis

- Other types of meningitis.
- Meningism (symptoms with normal CSF) associated with systemic illness.
- Subarachnoid haemorrhage.

Diagnosis

- Blood cultures are usually positive.
- Lumbar puncture is carried out providing there is no evidence of raised intracranial pressure. The CSF pressure is increased. A raised CSF protein (>0.4 g/l), polymorphs (>4/mm^3) and low glucose (<2/3 of serum glucose) will be found. Gram staining: Gram-positive cocci (*S. pneumoniae*, Group B streptococci), Gram-negative diplococci (*N. meningitidis*), Gram-negative bacilli or coccobacilli (*E. coli*, *H. influenzae*), Gram-positive bacilli (*L. monocytogenes*). CSF culture will confirm the diagnosis.
- A raised white cell count on blood film is indicative.
- Bacterial antigens may be detected in CSF or blood.

Treatment

- If the diagnosis is suspected, especially in the presence of a rash, parenteral penicillin should be administered (20–40 mg/kg) before transfer to hospital.
- Appropriate early therapy is cefotaxime, or other third-generation cephalosporins, in the neonate and child under 5 years. Children under 5 years may also be given chloramphenicol with or without benzylpenicillin. For children over the age of 5 years, chloramphenicol, cefotaxime or benzylpenicillin is appropriate. All should be given iv.
- When the causative organism has been identified, the most suitable treatment is cefotaxime 30–50 mg/kg, 8 hourly, for *E. coli* or *H. influenzae*, benzylpenicillin 20–40 mg/kg, 4–6 hourly, for Group B streptococci, *S. pneumoniae* and *N. meningitidis*, chloramphenicol 12–15 mg/kg, 6 hourly, for *H. influenzae* and *L. monocytogenes*. *Listeria* may also respond to ampicillin 15 mg/kg, 6 hourly, with gentamicin 11–17 mg/kg, 8 hourly.
- Steroids may have a role in the treatment of children.

Prevention

- All close household and kissing contacts of patients with *N. meningitidis* should receive rifampicin 600 mg twice a day for 2 days

(10 mg/kg for children over 1 year of age). Ciprofloxacin may also be used but in adults only.

- Similar prophylaxis but for 4 days should be given to contacts of *H. influenzae* cases under 5 years old and their parents.
- There is a vaccine for Groups A and C meningococci.

Aseptic meningitis

Aseptic meningitis is the term used to describe a syndrome of subacute onset of meningism with a lymphocytic CSF.

Causative agents

- Viruses (e.g. enterocytopathogenic human orphan [ECHO], Coxsackie and mumps).
- Bacteria (*L. monocytogenes*, *Mycobacterium tuberculosis*).
- Cerebral abscess.
- Fungi (*Cryptococcus neoformans*).
- Non-infective causes (malignancies) may be found.

Epidemiology and pathophysiology

- Mumps meningitis can occur with or without parotitis.
- Enterovirus infections (ECHO and Coxsackie) are seen in summer epidemics.
- Listeria (*see* acute bacterial meningitis, page 7).
- Tuberculous meningitis is most common in ethnic minorities (Asian and African), the elderly, alcoholics and the immunocompromised.
- Cases of viral meningitis outnumber those of bacterial meningitis by about 10:1.

Incubation period

- Mumps: 14–28 days.
- Enterovirus: 5 days.

Clinical features

- Symptoms are similar to those of acute bacterial meningitis but usually much less severe. Neck stiffness may be present only on extreme flexion.
- Tuberculous meningitis often causes headache and low-grade fever without neck stiffness in the early stages.

Differential diagnosis

- *See* acute bacterial meningitis (page 7).
- Lumbar puncture should be carried out. In viral meningitis CSF pressure is normal or mildly raised (4–30 cm H_2O), protein raised (0.4–1 g/l), glucose normal (>2/3 serum glucose), cells, mainly lymphocytes (>4/mm³). In tuberculous meningitis, the CSF pressure is usually high, the protein sometimes very high (>1 g/l), glucose low and organisms may be seen using auramine or Ziehl–Nielsen staining.
- Viruses may be isolated from throat, stool or CSF samples.

Treatment

- Viral meningitis, once confirmed, is treated with rest and analgesics.
- Other infections require appropriate antibiotics (*see* tuberculosis, page 41).

Prevention

- The mumps component of the mumps, measles and rubella (MMR) vaccine will effectively prevent this disease.
- Tuberculous meningitis may be prevented by inoculation with bacillus Calmette Guérin (BCG) vaccine. Close contacts of open pulmonary TB should be closely monitored (*see* tuberculosis, page 41).

Encephalitis

Causative agents

- A wide range of viruses, including herpes simplex virus (HSV), varicella zoster and enteroviruses.
- Non-viral infective agents including *Mycoplasma*, *L. monocytogenes*, Lyme disease, *Brucella*, and *Toxoplasma* in the immunocompromised.
- Post-infective encephalomyelitis occurs following specific viral infections, such as measles, rubella and chickenpox.
- Insect-borne viruses in various parts of the world, e.g. tick-borne encephalitis in Scandinavia.

Epidemiology

- The most serious form of encephalitis, that due to HSV, occurs at any time of year.
- Other causes can be related to the season and epidemic status.

Incubaton period

- In mumps, HSV and other infective agents, the invasion of the CNS by the virus often occurs simultaneously with other disease manifestations.
- Post-infective encephalomyelitis is seen up to 2 weeks after the initial infection.

Clinical features

- The major features are altered consciousness and fever, which may be low-grade.
- Meningism – fever, headache, nausea, neck stiffness – is common.
- Developing focal neurological signs and seizures are also common.
- Other signs of the infectious agent may be present, such as herpes labialis or the characteristic rash of chickenpox or measles.
- The clinical course varies, depending on the infectious agent and influence of therapy. Herpes simplex encephalitis is associated with a high (50%) mortality when untreated, and morbidity is common in the survivors, whereas chickenpox encephalitis has a much better prognosis in which death and long-term sequelae are uncommon.

Differential diagnosis

- Other causes of depressed consciousness, including drug overdose, head injury, hepatic failure, Reye's syndrome, legionnaires' disease and severe systemic illness in the elderly.
- Cerebral abscess.

Diagnosis

- The CSF changes are as those seen in aseptic meningitis.
- Specific cultures and antibody tests may retrospectively aid diagnosis of causes such as HSV and enterovirus.
- CT and electroencephalography (EEG) are frequently helpful, especially in the diagnosis of HSV infection.

Treatment

- For most causes, therapy involves supportive care only. Steroids and mannitol have a limited role.
- Acyclovir 10 mg/kg, 8 hourly, iv is of benefit in encephalitis due to HSV and varicella zoster (chickenpox).

- Specific antibiotic therapy is effective for the infrequent cases caused by bacteria, which, therefore, should be sought exhaustively.

Prevention

- None.

CHAPTER 3

Upper respiratory tract infections

WHILST the majority of these conditions are mild and self-limiting, they are some of the most frequent causes of illness and absenteeism from work. However, included in the differential diagnosis are some potentially serious infections. Most sore throats will be due to minor viral infection, but missing the occasional more aggressive disease, such as quinsy, diphtheria or anginose glandular fever can result in a marked increase in morbidity and mortality. Doctors should satisfy themselves that they understand the clinical differences enough to avoid the potential problems.

Streptococcal tonsillitis/pharyngitis

Causative agent

● *Streptococcus pyogenes* (Lancefield Group A β-haemolytic streptococcus).

Epidemiology and pathophysiology

● Droplet spread, although food and drink have also been implicated as sources.
● There are numerous serotypes based on the Griffith typing of M antigens.
● The organism can elaborate a number of toxins, including haemolysin, streptodornase, erythrogenic toxins, hyaluronidase and streptokinase.

Incubation period

● 1–4 days.

Clinical features

● The majority of infections are asymptomatic.
● When symptoms do occur, they vary from mild to severe and include fever (up to 40°C), pain on swallowing, tender cervical adenopathy, anorexia and malaise.

- Examination will reveal enlarged, tender cervical lymph nodes, especially just below the angle of the jaw (tonsillar nodes). The pharynx is diffusely red and the tonsils, if present, may have a punctate (follicular) white exudate.
- Complications include peritonsillar abscess (quinsy), septicaemia, scarlet fever, rheumatic fever, glomerulonephritis, erythema nodosum and erythema multiforme.

Differential diagnosis

- Epstein–Barr virus (EBV) infection.
- Throat infections caused by other viruses, which are usually milder and less often associated with exudative tonsillitis, although adeno-virus can cause a severe tonsillitis.
- Other causes of sore throat: herpangina, Vincent's angina, herpes simplex stomatitis, and oral candidiasis.

Diagnosis

- The diagnosis can be established in 24 hours by culture of a throat swab.
- An anti-streptolysin 'O' titre when seen to rise in serial blood samples will retrospectively confirm the diagnosis.
- A neutrophil leucocytosis can be seen on blood film.

Treatment

- Penicillin V 7 mg/kg orally, 6 hourly, or erythromycin at the same dose for 10 days is usually effective. Parenteral therapy is required in severe cases.
- Ampicillin, amoxycillin or pivampicillin should never be given, because of the possibility of EBV infection as a cause of the symptoms. Such patients almost invariably develop an unpleasant rash and fever, but there is no lasting hypersensitivity to those drugs.

Prevention

- In the rare patient prone to rheumatic fever, long-term penicillin (at least 5 years) is given as daily oral doses or monthly injections.

Epstein–Barr virus (glandular fever, infectious mononucleosis)

Causative agent

- EBV, a herpes virus that infects epithelial and lymphoid tissue.

Epidemiology

- Infection is common, although usually asymptomatic in children.
- Symptoms more commonly occur in young adults.
- The mode of transmission is by droplet spread, kissing and sexual contact.
- The incidence of symptomatic disease is approximately 207 cases per 100 000 population per year in England and Wales.
- 30% of children have been infected by the age of 5 years.
- Twice as many cases occur in the autumn and winter as in the spring and summer.
- The infection has been linked to Burkitt's and other lymphomas, nasopharyngeal carcinomas and oral hairy leukoplakia.

Incubation period

- 10–50 days.

Clinical features

- Symptoms include tiredness, sore throat, malaise, headache, and fever, which varies between mild and very high.
- Tonsillitis is common (30%), with a characteristic cream/yellow confluent exudate and palatal petechiae, although the majority (85%) have a sore throat.
- Lymphadenopathy, which is mainly cervical but also involves other regions, is found in 95%, and is only very mildly tender.
- Splenomegaly is felt in 50%.
- Rash in glandular fever is quite rare except a severe maculopapular, measles-like eruption associated with amoxycillin, pivampicillin and ampicillin. There is no lasting hypersensitivity to these drugs.
- The most severe consequence of this disease is respiratory obstruction due to pharyngeal oedema and tonsillar hypertrophy.
- Icteric hepatitis may occur in about 10% of cases with features similar to other viral hepatitides, and often has cholestatic features with a raised alkaline phosphatase.

- The disease usually persists for only 2–3 weeks and then gradually subsides, although fatigue and malaise may last for much longer.
- The disease occasionally presents with fever alone (<5%).
- Complications can include prolonged debility, cold-agglutinin haemolytic anaemia, traumatic splenic rupture, thombocytopenic purpura, meningitis, encephalomyelitis, polyneuritis or mono-neuritis, and myocarditis or pericarditis.

Differential diagnosis

- A peripheral blood picture demonstrates atypical lymphocytes in 70% of cases usually representing 10–25% of the differential count, with an associated lymphocytosis, and neutropenia.
- The Paul–Bunnell test or monospot tests for heterophile antibodies are positive in the acute stage in 90% of cases, and this result persists for about 1 year. The test may be negative at first, but it is worth repeating it if the diagnosis is strongly suspected.
- The results of liver function tests are commonly abnormal, in particular a raised alanine transferase.
- Alkaline phosphatase and bilirubin may also be raised during the hepatitis.
- IgG and IgM antibodies to the EBV capsular antigen (VCA) and nuclear antigen (EBNA) can establish a diagnosis in the 10% of patients who are monospot-negative.

Treatment

- Treatment is mainly symptomatic.
- Steroids may be appropriate in patients in whom the exudative tonsil-litis and pharyngitis are so severe that they may begin to threaten the airway, when difficulty in swallowing and speaking will be present.
- Steroids may also be given for the haemolytic anaemia, or for very prolonged and severe acute attacks.

Prevention

- There is no vaccine.
- As asymptomatic disease is the most likely outcome of infection, isolation is unnecessary.

Diphtheria

Causative agent

- *Corynebacterium diphtheriae.*

Epidemiology

- A disease mainly affecting children 2–14 years of age.
- The organism is droplet spread.
- There are three biotypes: mitis, intermedius and gravis, given in order of increasing severity.
- It is now extremely rare in the developed world although still common in developing countries. There were 2 recorded cases in the UK in 1987.
- Asymptomatic throat carriage is common in endemic areas.

Incubation period

- 2–4 days.

Clinical features

- The manifestations are due to both infection and toxin production.
- Infection can be limited to the nose with a clear, purulent or bloody discharge.
- Throat infection is marked by sudden onset of fever (up to 39°C), sore throat and malaise. The pharynx is red with an initially clear, shiny membrane on the tonsils, uvula, palate or pharynx. Over subsequent days, this becomes grey and often black with underlying haemorrhage. There is often extensive swelling of the cervical lymph nodes ('bull neck'). The larger the membrane, the more ill the patient.
- Extension of infection to the larynx leads to hoarse voice, stridor, coarse cough and eventual severe respiratory obstruction, which requires tracheotomy.
- Toxin production leads to heart and nervous system disease.
- Cardiac dysfunction develops in 10–25% of cases 1–2 weeks after infection. The cardiotoxin induces conduction defects and myocarditis, leading to cardiac failure and circulatory collapse. There is a high mortality, particularly in association with atrioventricular (AV) block. These changes can be permanent.
- Neurotoxin damage, as with cardiotoxin effects, is proportional to the severity of infection. Palatal and pharyngeal paralysis is commonly the first sign and occurs early in the infection. Cranial nerve palsies may follow with peripheral neuropathies developing 1–12 weeks later. Motor or mixed motor/sensory proximal or distal neuropathies occur. This is slowly reversible. Up to 75% of cases of severe infection will have associated neurological disease.
- Cutaneous infection is seen occasionally in the tropics.

Differential diagnosis

- All other causes of pharyngitis.

Diagnosis

- Diagnosis is essentially clinical from recognition of the membrane, nasal discharge, toxicity out of proportion to the fever, and respiratory involvement.
- Confirmation comes from a throat swab inoculated onto Loeffler's serum medium or tellurite medium, speciation of the organism and confirmation of toxin production.

Treatment

- After ensuring that the airway is protected, the patient should be transferred to an isolation unit and diphtheria antitoxin up to 100 000 units administered as soon as possible.
- Benzylpenicillin 13 mg/kg, 6 hourly, iv or erythromycin, 7 mg/kg, 6 hourly for 14 days will being rapid resolution in uncomplicated cases.
- Supportive care is required for cardiac and nervous disease and for the severely ill patient.

Prevention

- The falling incidence of this disease is related to a very effective vaccine (diphtheria toxoid, see Chapter 17) and to a better standard of living.
- The Schick test, which depends on antibody neutralization of intradermally injected toxin, may indicate the immune status of individuals at risk of exposure.
- Antibiotic prophylaxis with penicillin or erythromycin can be given to those contacts of cases who may not be immune.
- The index case should receive immunization because natural infection does not confer immunity.

Oral ulceration

Causative agents

- HSV type I.
- Enteroviruses.
- Varicella zoster virus.
- *Borrelia vincentii* with *Fusobacterium nucleatum* (Vincent's organisms).
- Drugs.

Epidemiology

- Viral causes are spread by droplets or kissing.
- Vincent's organisms are oral commensals.
- HSV infects at least 50% of the population, most of whom acquire the infection by puberty.

Incubation period

- Primary HSV: 2–12 days.
- Enteroviruses: 2–10 days.
- Varicella zoster: 7–23 days.

Clinical features

- Mouth ulcers frequently present with localized pain, which is often associated with cervical adenopathy and fever. In the majority of cases, the correct aetiological diagnosis can be made from the characteristic associated features.
- HSV is often asymptomatic but may present in children under the age of 5 years as gingivostomatitis. Multiple small vesicles rapidly rupture to leave extensive small painful ulcers, which may coalesce, on the tongue, lips, gums palate, buccal mucosa and pharynx. There is an associated fever (up to 39°C) and tender cervical adenopathy. The child is frequently unable to swallow during the 10–14-day illness. Recurrence of infection is usually confined to discrete herpes labialis ('cold sores') although HSV pharyngitis has been described. Herpes labialis is a reactivation of virus harboured in dorsal route ganglia and induced by stress of various types.
- There are two enterovirus-related syndromes in which oral ulceration is characteristic. Herpangina is a shortlived Coxsackie virus infection of children in which fever and cervical adenopathy are associated with multiple small vesicles and ulcers on the soft palate, uvula, tonsils and pharynx. Hand, foot and mouth disease, due to Coxsackie A16, also primarily affects children under 10 years. The multiple small painful ulcers and vesicles are seen mainly on the tongue and buccal mucosa, in association with fever and a rash on the hands and feet, which is vesicular or papular. Both conditions are common but mild, and rarely last more than 7 days.
- Acute necrotizing ulcerative gingivitis (ANUG), due to synergistic infection with *Borrelia vincentii* and *Fusobacterium nucleatum*, is a condition seen at any age in which painful ulceration and inflammation of the gingival mucosa develops suddenly and severely. The ulcerated gums bleed easily and there is a characteristic halitosis, often

with fever and cervical adenopathy. Antibiotic and local antiseptic treatment is curative, but the untreated case may progress to more extensive oral and pharyngeal disease (Vincent's angina) or rarely to a widespread necrosis of the mouth and oral cavity (cancrum oris).

● Aphthous ulceration is a condition of unknown cause in which painful ulcers appear singly or in small numbers on the mouth and buccal mucosa, particularly at times of stress. These may occasionally be associated with systemic disease such as Crohn's disease and Behçet's syndrome.

● Oral ulceration can occur during chickenpox, facial shingles, and Stevens–Johnson syndrome, in which cases the diagnosis is obvious from the rash.

Diagnosis

● Diagnosis can be made from the constellation of associated features.
● HSV and enterovirus infections can be confirmed by tissue culture of throat swab specimens transported in appropriate medium.
● Vincent's organisms will be seen on Gram staining of a smear taken from the inflamed gum.

Treatment

● HSV responds to acyclovir 3 mg/kg 5 times daily for 5 days. This may be given prophylactically for frequent recurrence of herpes labialis. Topical acyclovir cream will cure uncomplicated herpes labialis.
● ANUG clears rapidly after dilute hydrogen peroxide mouthwashes and either penicillin V 7 mg/kg, 6 hourly, or metronidazole 3 mg/kg, 8 hourly, for 1 week.

Prevention

● HSV infection in children can be avoided if adults with herpes labialis desist from kissing the youngsters during an acute attack.

Oral candidiasis (thrush)

Causative agent

● *Candida albicans*.

Epidemiology

● A saprophytic commensal yeast commonly found in the mouth, vagina and intestine without causing infection.

● Predisposing factors making candida infection more likely are pregnancy, diabetes mellitus, the oral contraceptive pill, long-term use of steroids, antibiotics, immunosuppression and AIDS.

Incubation period

● Occurs 1–2 weeks after antibiotic therapy commences.

Clinical features

● The patient complains of a sore mouth, in which plaques are seen on the palate and tongue. These can be removed to reveal a haemorrhagic base.

Differential diagnosis

● Mucus or food adhering to the mouth can be mistaken for candida.

Diagnosis

● The organism is readily recognized on clinical grounds, but can easily be seen with direct microscopy of a suitable sample.

Treatment

● Oral thrush responds readily to nystatin suspension, amphotericin lozenges or fluconazole capsules, in resistant recurring cases.

Prevention

● Antibiotics should be given only when bacterial infection is likely, thus reducing the incidence of thrush as a side-effect.
● Patients on inhaled steroids should rinse out their mouth after use.

Common cold (coryza)

Causative agents

● A large number of viruses of the myxovirus, paramyxovirus, adenovirus, picornavirus and coronavirus groups.

Epidemiology

- The majority of cases are seen between September and March.
- In peak months, 0.6–0.8% of the population will be infected at any one time.
- Transmission is mainly by droplet, hand-to-hand and hand-to-nose spread.
- Children act as reservoirs and introduce the infection into the home where there will be a variable number of secondary cases.

Incubation period

- Mainly 2–5 days.

Clinical features

- Nasal discharge and obstruction, sore throat, cough and mild fever are the main symptoms.
- The illness lasts for 1–2 weeks, although respiratory syncytial virus infections can last for up to 4 weeks.
- Complications are few, but include sinusitis, nose bleeds, lower respiratory tract infections and otitis media.

Differential diagnosis

- This syndrome can be seen as part of the illness in streptococcal pharyngitis, measles, diphtheria, influenza and mycoplasma infections.
- Hayfever and other types of rhinitis can cause diagnostic difficulties.

Diagnosis

- Diagnosis is almost invariably clinical.
- Virological diagnosis is rarely helpful or necessary.

Treatment

- Symptomatic relief with analgesics, nasal decongestants and antihistamines.
- Although antiviral agents, such as nasal sprays of alpha-interferon, are effective in the early phase, they are not of practical use.

Prevention

- There are too many viruses for possible vaccine development.
- Isolation of index cases may be effective but it is rarely practical.

Sinusitis

Causative agents

● Acute sinusitis: mainly *S. pneumoniae, H. influenzae* and anaerobes.
● Chronic sinusitis: anaerobes.

Epidemiology

● Occurs as a complication of approximately 0.5% of common cold infections and is more frequent in people who have been swimming.
● It is most common in adults.

Incubation period

● 1–7 days from the onset of coryza.

Clinical features

● Any of the paranasal (frontal, maxillary or ethmoid) sinuses can become acutely infected.
● Often following, or during, a cold, the patient develops local facial pain, usually with nasal congestion, purulent nasal discharge and low-grade fever. There may be localized tenderness, erythema and oedema over the infected sinus.
● Recurrent attacks can occur.
● Complications include orbital cellulitis, facial osteomyelitis, meningitis and brain abscess.

Differential diagnosis

● The distinction from severe coryza is not always easy.

Diagnosis

● X-rays using specific sinus views will show opacification of fluid levels.
● Microbial identification is impossible without sinus puncture.

Treatment

● Antibiotics to cover the possible organisms empirically, such as amoxycillin or co-trimoxazole for 10 days, will be effective in the majority of cases.

- Amoxycillin and clavulanate (Augmentin) is useful for resistant acute cases and chronic infections.
- Nasal decongestants offer temporary symptomatic relief. Occasionally, surgical intervention is required for the more chronic cases when sinus drainage has become the major problem.

Prevention

- Antibiotics given during coryza attacks will not prevent sinusitis, but prompt treatment of acute sinusitis will prevent complications and reduce the risk of chronicity.

Influenza

Causative agent

- Influenza virus types A, B, and C each possess different characteristics. Type C is probably the least serious and Type A the most virulent.

Epidemiology and pathophysiology

- Droplet spread.
- The organisms possess haemagglutinin (H) and neuraminidase (N) antigens which can change gradually (antigenic drift) or suddenly (antigenic shift) within the population.
- Epidemics and pandemics are related to both antigenic shift and antigenic drift introducing new strains into a non-immune population.
- In the influenza epidemic that began in November 1989, there were 600 deaths in the UK attributed to it. In major epidemics, the number of deaths can rise to 20 000.
- Of all deaths, 82% occur in the over-65 years age-group.

Incubation period

- 1–5 days.

Clinical features

- Mild influenza may be difficult to distinguish from other upper respiratory tract infections, although the former usually starts abruptly and is likely to include several of the following symptoms: fever (up to 40°C), headache, vomiting, aching limbs and back, non-productive cough, muscle weakness and runny nose.

● The illness rarely lasts more than 5 days.
● Complications include pneumonia (viral or secondary bacterial), otitis media, sinusitis and depression.
● Each strain is typed according to antigen and named according to year and site of first identification, e.g. A/Taiwan/85/H1N1.
● The cause of antigenic variation is unknown, but may relate to novel virus strains introduced from other animals, such as pigs.

Differential diagnosis

● Lobar pneumonia.
● Viral meningitis.
● Pyelonephritis.
● Severe viral upper respiratory infections.

Diagnosis

● Diagnosis is usually clinical, although serology can be useful: a rise in titre in paired sera confirming infection.
● The virus can be grown from naso-pharyngeal swabs or aspurates.

Treatment

● Treatment is mainly supportive, apart from the treatment of specific complications. Amantadine given within the first day or two of the illness may reduce the severity of infections with influenza A but not B.
● Pneumonia presents with a sudden worsening of symptoms and is treated with antibiotics appropriate to the cause which is usually one of: *S. pneumoniae*, *H. influenzae*, *S. pyogenes* and *Staph. aureus*.

Prevention

● Avoidance of exposure is virtually impossible, particularly during epidemics.
● Vaccination is between 70 and 90% effective and should be offered to those at particular risk: the elderly, patients with chronic cardio-vascular, respiratory or renal disease, diabetes or other endocrine diseases and immunocompromised patients.
● The vaccine is effective between 1 and 3 weeks after immunization.

- Allergy to eggs is a contraindication to vaccination.
- A different vaccine is required each year because of the changing strains.

Croup/laryngitis/epiglottitis

Causative agents

- A variety of viruses including para-influenza, influenza, respiratory syncytial and enteroviruses.
- *H. influenzae* causes epiglottitis in the age-group less than 5 years old.

Epidemiology

- These diseases are seen mainly in the colder months.
- They are all droplet spread.
- Laryngitis afflicts people of any age, whereas croup and epiglottitis are seen in children below the age of 5 years.

Incubation period

- Usually 2–5 days.

Clinical features

- All three diseases characteristically present with coryzal symptoms and fever in association with a hoarse voice and barking cough.
- Croup (laryngotracheobronchitis) is a disease of viral aetiology where there is additionally a stridor (inspiratory wheeze) and mild-to-moderate respiratory distress. The fever is rarely higher than 38°C, and the child is not usually toxic.
- Acute epiglottitis, usually related to capsulated *H. influenzae*, causes abrupt high fever, severe constitutional upset and a stridor which can vary markedly with position. The inflamed epiglottis can suddenly obstruct the larnyx making this disease a medical emergency.
- Laryngitis and croup usually improve in 1–7 days, although croup often recurs in subsequent viral infections.

Differential diagnosis

- Inhaled foreign bodies should be excluded in children.
- Epiglottitis is usually more severe, but clinical differentiation can be very difficult.

Diagnosis

- Lateral soft-tissue X-ray of the neck is diagnostic. The throat should not be examined, as this may precipitate respiratory obstruction.

Treatment

- Laryngitis requires symptomatic treatment and voice rest.
- Croup may, in addition, improve with air humidification. Occasional very severe cases require steroids and sometimes temporary intubation of the airway.
- Epiglottitis is treated with parenteral chloramphenicol 7 mg/kg, 6 hourly, or cefotaxime 30 mg/kg, 8 hourly, in a unit where intubation or tracheostomy is immediately available if respiratory arrest ensues. The infection resolves within 5 days of treatment.

Prevention

- None of these diseases is preventable, except in close household contacts of severe disease caused by *H. influenzae*. These may be given prophylactic rifampicin 20 mg/kg twice for 4 days.

Ear infections

Causative agents

Otitis media
- Mainly *S. pneumoniae* and *H. influenzae*.
- Also *Moraxella (Branhamella) catarrhalis* and *S. pyogenes*.

Otitis externa
- *Staph. aureus*.
- Gram-negative bacilli, especially *Pseudomonas aeruginosa* (particularly in the 'malignant' type).

Epidemiology

- Otitis media is mainly a disease of pre-school children, but it can occur at any age. It seems to be related to poor drainage of the middle ear by the Eustachian tube.
- Otitis externa occurs at any age and is often related to swimming, hot humid weather, recurrent otitis media and a narrow external auditory canal.

Incubation period

- Unknown, although acute otitis externa can occur 1–3 days after swimming.

Clinical features

- Otitis media produces a rapid onset of fever and severe ear pain. The child is distressed and often tugs at the ear lobe. Spontaneous rupture of the tympanic membrane brings rapid improvement. The tympanic membrane will be seen on auroscopy to be red, immobile and lacking a light reflex.
- Otitis externa can be acute in onset, with a pustule seen in the external auditory canal ('acute localized'), or erythema and oedema of the canal and pinna ('acute diffuse'). Chronic otitis externa is a condition in which the inflamed canal is filled with purulent exudate from middle-ear disease. A 'malignant' form is seen in the elderly and diabetics, in which there is a chronic spreading infection to adjacent tissues with associated necrosis.
- Otitis media can lead to mastoiditis acutely, and recurrent attacks may lead to glue ear (secretory otitis media) and hearing difficulties.

Differential diagnosis

- Many conditions are associated with a mildly red tympanic membrane, including measles and influenza, but treatment is not required.
- In otitis externa, especially in children, an impacted foreign body must be excluded.

Diagnosis

- Diagnosis is entirely clinical for otitis media, but bacterial swabs of the exudate in otitis externa can guide treatment.

Treatment

- There is debate about the use of antibiotics in otitis media. Many recent trials suggest that simple analgesics alone give an identical result. Myringotomy may be required for symptomatic relief in indolent cases.
- Localized otitis externa requires analgesia alone, whereas diffuse otitis externa requires cleansing with an antiseptic solution followed by antibiotic eardrops, although systemic antibiotics may be required.

Therapy of chronic otitis externa depends on antibiotics for the underlying otitis media. Malignant otitis externa is best dealt with surgically and with antipseudomonal agents.
● Complicating mastoiditis, identified by swelling and pain in the area behind the ear, requires vigorous antibiotic therapy.

Prevention

● Of these conditions, only otitis externa in swimmers may be prevented by the use of ear plugs and scrupulous drying of the external auditory canal.

CHAPTER 4

Lower respiratory tract infections

THE majority of these infections are serious and frequently life-threatening. The initial diagnosis is important as most of these patients will require in-patient care, except, perhaps, for some of those with an exacerbation of chronic bronchitis or the mildest of the lobar pneumonias. In this section, the aim is to enable the doctor to come to an aetiological diagnosis at an early stage, thus allowing appropriate initial therapy.

Community-acquired acute pneumonias in adults

Causative agents

- *S. pneumoniae* (40–50%).
- *Mycoplasma pneumoniae* (10–20%).
- *Legionella pneumophila* (5–10%).
- Other causes include *Chlamydia psittaci* (psittacosis), *Coxiella burnetii* (Q fever), *Staph. aureus*, *S. pyogenes*, *Klebsiella pneumoniae*, influenza and respiratory syncytial viruses (RSVs).

Epidemiology

- *See* separate organisms.

Incubation periods

- *See* separate organisms.

Clinical features

- The characteristic features of acute pneumonia are fever, cough, dyspnoea and, occasionally, pleuritic pain. Examination may reveal a dull percussion note over the consolidated area, where bronchial breathing, inspiratory fine crackles, decreased breathing sounds and a plural rub may be heard. These symptoms and signs are variable, and acute pneumonia may present with fever in the absence of symptoms or signs referrable to the chest.
- It is often possible to come to an aetiological diagnosis on clinical grounds.

- Acute pneumococcal pneumonia presents with sudden onset of high fever (up to 40°C), a dry or sparsely productive cough, occasionally 'rusty' sputum or pleuritic pain. Chest signs may be discrete but can include those of a pleural effusion in addition to the ones described above. Herpes labialis is often present.
- *Mycoplasma pneumoniae* spreads by droplet and within families with an incubation period of 15–25 days. As well as pneumonia, there may be several people afflicted with a 'flu-like illness. The pneumonia has a subacute onset, and several days of increasingly severe symptoms usually preceding the illness for which the patient seeks medical attention. Fever is most usually in the range of 38–39°C associated with a dry or mildly productive cough, but pleuritic pain is unusual. Physical signs of consolidation can be completely absent and, in association with frequently extensive chest X-ray changes, have led to the appellation 'primary atypical pneumonia'.
- Legionnaires' disease is acquired when *Legionella pneumophila*, a Gram-negative bacillus, is allowed to grow in warm (<60°C) man-made water systems and is aerosolized. Such situations occur in roof-top air conditioning cooling towers associated with appropriate wind conditions, showers and poorly plumbed hot-water systems. Outbreaks occur in the UK when cooling towers are poorly maintained, and in foreign hotels when holidaymakers shower in luke-warm water. The pneumonia is mainly seen in the elderly, smokers and the immunocompromised. Some people undergo a 'flu-like illness ('Pontiac fever') when exposed. After a 2–10-day incubation period, the onset can be identical to pneumococcal pneumonia. This multisystem disease also has associated symptoms of diarrhoea (50%), nausea/vomiting and abdominal pain (20%), confusion (20–50%) and, less commonly, jaundice and anuria. Some cases present with confusion or 'gastroenteritis' as the sole symptoms other than fever. The disease has a 10% fatality rate.
- There are two further 'primary atypical pneumonias', one due to *Chlamydia psittaci* (psittacosis) and the other to *Coxiella burnetii* (Q fever). Both conditions present in an almost identical fashion to mycoplasma pneumonia. However, epidemiological features may point to the diagnosis. Psittacosis occurs after contact with infected birds, mainly pigeons or budgerigars and parrots, with an incubation period of 4–28 days. Q fever is also a disease of domestic animals and is more likely to occur in farmers, abattoir workers and visitors to the Mediterranean, being transmitted by contact with animals, animal products and by tick-bites. The incubation period is 14–28 days. Both organisms can also have renal and hepatic effects, and *Coxiella burnetii* is also a significant cause of infective endocarditis.

- The pneumonias caused by *Klebsiella pneumoniae* and *Staph. aureus* are very similar, both causing a severe illness, often with multiple lung abscess formation. They occur mainly in the debilitated host: *Klebsiella* affecting alcoholics, diabetics, and chronic bronchitis sufferers, and the staphylococcus in the setting of influenza and other viral infections, iv drug abuse and aspiration. Their presentation is usually similar to pneumococcal pneumonia although purulent or blood-stained sputum is more common. Mortality is high.
- The pneumonias associated with respiratory syncytial virus and, particularly, influenza can be viral or bacterial. Viral pneumonia is a smooth progression from the initial upper respiratory infection in a child or elderly patient. Bacterial pneumonia presents as a sudden deterioration in the course of illness with increase in fever and cough. In this situation, the most likely organisms are *S. pneumoniae, Staph. aureus, S. pyogenes* and *H. influenzae*.

Differential diagnosis

- Differentiating mild pneumonia from severe bronchitis can depend on the chest X-ray.
- When the chest symptoms and signs are subtle, the disease can be similar to a wide range of other febrile illnesses.
- Other chest infections such as TB and bronchiectasis can also be manifest in similar ways.

Diagnosis

- The diagnosis of pneumonia rests on the chest X-ray. In all except viral causes, lobar or lobular consolidation will be seen. *Mycoplasma, Chlamydia* and *Coxiella* may also cause multiple lobe involvement or a diffuse pneumonitis, the latter also being seen in viral pneumonia.
- A white cell count on the blood film can be very helpful. In primary viral, legionella, chlamydia, coxiella and myoplasma pneumonias the white count is normal or only mildly raised ($<15 \times 10^9$/l). Lymphopenia is also seen with *Legionella*.
- In legionnaires' disease, hyponatraemia, in addition to abnormal renal and liver function tests, is a frequent finding.
- Confirmation of cause can be made through sputum culture and blood culture for the bacterial infections. The rest are diagnosed serologically (immunofluorescent or complement fixation antibody tests). *Legionella* can be stained in the sputum and will grow on special media, although the immunofluorescent antibody test is most often used. The virus may be grown from throat swabs in appropriate transport medium.

Treatment

- Some pneumonias can be managed at home.
- When the cause is unknown, the most effective antibiotic is erythromycin 7 mg/kg, 6 hourly. If staphylococci or *Klebsiella* are a likely cause, chloramphenicol 7 mg/kg, 6 hourly, may be given.
- Specific treatments would be benzylpenicillin 20–50 mg/kg, 6 hourly (*S. pneumoniae*), erythromycin 7 mg/kg, 6 hourly (*S. pneumoniae*, *Mycoplasma*, *Coxiella*, *Chlamydia* and *Legionella*). *Legionella* may not respond to erythromycin alone, in which case rifampicin 10 mg/kg, 12 hourly, is added. Staphylococcal pneumonia is best treated with flucloxacillin 7–30 mg/kg, 6 hourly, to which fusidic acid or rifampicin may be added. Klebsiella pneumonia responds to therapy with a third-generation cephalosporin or aminoglycoside given iv.
- Primary viral pneumonia responds poorly to therapy although nebulized ribavirin has been used for RSV infection with some success in children.

Prevention

- Pneumococcal vaccine is of relatively low efficacy, but may be offered to those at high risk of such infection, e.g. patients about to undergo splenectomy.

Childhood pneumonias

Causative agents

- Neonates: *E. coli*, other Gram-negative bacilli, Lancefield Group B streptococci and *Chlamydia trachomatis*.
- Children under 5 years of age: *H. influenzae*, *S. pneumoniae*, *Mycoplasma pneumoniae*, RSV.

Epidemiology

- *See* individual organisms.

Incubation period

- *See* individual organisms.

Clinical features

● Neonatal pneumonia presents with respiratory distress, fever and failure to thrive. The infecting organisms are acquired from the mother, and the infection presents within the first week of life. Nursery outbreaks of *Chlamydia* have been recorded. A chest X-ray is routinely taken of all neonates who are ill, because physical signs specific to pneumonia are usually absent.

● Pneumonia in the under 5-year-old is most usually non-specific in its presentation, except that it may be preceded by a specific viral infection, such as measles or influenza. In the case of an H. influenzae aetiology the onset can be insidious, over several days; a more sudden onset occurs with *S. pneumoniae*. Fever is invariably present although dyspnoea and cough less so; other symptoms seen frequently include vomiting and diarrhoea. Physical signs of consolidation are often subtle or absent. Complications include pleural effusion, septicaemia and the other distant infective manifestations of these organisms such as meningitis.

● The clinical features of infection with *Mycoplasma pneumoniae* are similar to those with H. influenzae pneumonia, often preceded by an upper respiratory infection. Haemolytic anaemia is a rare complication.

● RSV pneumonia is indistinguishable from acute bronchiolitis clinically (*see* bronchiolitis, page 37).

Differential diagnosis

● The symptoms and signs are often non-specific. In this case, meningitis, urinary tract infection and gastroenteritis are also possible.

● Non-infective chest problems, including inhaled foreign body and asthma, can be similar in presentation.

● Mild pneumonia may be clinically indistinguishable from acute bronchitis.

Diagnosis

● Neonatal pneumonia causes lobar or patchy consolidation.

● The chest X-ray shows lobar consolidation in infections with *H. influenzae*, *S. pneumoniae* and *Mycoplasma pneumoniae*, although the first two agents may produce the widespread patchy changes of bronchopneumonia. Diffuse interstitial changes may be seen in pneumonias caused by *Mycoplasma pneumoniae* and RSV.

- Blood and sputum culture, if obtainable, may provide a specific diagnosis of neonatal bacterial pathogens, *S. pneumoniae* and *H. influenzae*. *Mycoplasma pneumoniae* is diagnosed serologically (immunofluorescent antibody test) and RSV from culture of nasal secretions.
- Cold agglutinins are present in the blood of about 50% of people with mycoplasma infections.

Treatment

- Neonatal infections are treated with a third-generation cephalosporin or erythromycin if *Chlamydia* is the pathogen.
- Beyond the neonatal period, erythromycin 7 mg/kg, 6 hourly, is effective for the majority of bacterial pathogens although *H. influenzae* may be resistant. Benzylpenicillin 20–50 mg/kg, 6 hourly (*S. pneumoniae*) and cefotaxime 15–30 mg/kg, 8 hourly, or co-trimoxazole (5 mg/kg of trimethoprim), 12 hourly (*H. influenzae*) are suitable specific therapies. Mycoplasma responds to erythromycin as above, and RSV may respond to nebulized ribavirin.

Prevention

- Neonatal infection may be anticipated by the isolation of *Chlamydia* and Group B streptococci from the maternal genital tract.
- Rifampicin 20 mg/kg, daily, for 4 days may be given to under 5-year-old household contacts and their parents, of cases infected with *H. influenzae*.

Infective exacerbations of cystic fibrosis, chronic bronchitis and bronchopneumonia

Causative agents

- Commonly, *S. pneumoniae*, *H. influenzae*, with *Pseudomonas* sp. in cystic fibrosis.
- Occasionally, *Pseudomonas aeruginosa* (chronic bronchitis) and *Moraxella (Branhamella) catarrhalis*.

Epidemiology and pathophysiology

- Cystic fibrosis is a congenital disease of mucus secretion causing airways damage in children and young adults, with associated abnormalities in pancreatic function.

- Frequent acute chest infections are seen in the background of chronic colonization of the airways with *Pseudomonas aeruginosa* in a large proportion of cases.
- Chronic bronchitis and emphysema are diseases mainly of adulthood resulting from chronic airways damage, due to factors such as smoking and asthma.
- Recurrent chest infections, often precipitated by a viral illness, are common.
- Bronchopneumonia may result from infection in these two conditions, or may arise afresh as a result of infection with more potent pathogens in the normal lung.

Incubation period

- The bacterial infections are generally not transmissible, but often arise from chronic carriage.

Clinical features

- The infective exacerbations of chronic bronchitis and cystic fibrosis may start with a viral upper respiratory infection, although many are undoubtedly related to a primary infection with the bacterial pathogen. There is a rise in temperature with an increase in production of yellow sputum, worsening dyspnoea and wheezing.
- There are no clinically distinguishing features between infective bronchitis and subsequent bronchopneumonia, except for more severe symptoms in the latter.
- Patients with cystic fibrosis almost invariably become colonized with *Pseudomonas aeruginosa*. There is still debate regarding the pathogenicity of the organism in this setting, although most physicians use antibiotics to suppress the infection.
- Complications of infection include lung abscess, emphysema, septicaemia and embolic infection.

Differential diagnosis

- The distinguishing feature between bronchitis and bronchopneumonia is the presence of widespread patchy consolidation on the chest X-ray.
- Culture of sputum and, rarely, blood will usually identify the responsible organism.

Treatment

- Therapy with any one of the many broad-spectrum antibiotics can be used including cephalosporins, co-trimoxazole, erythromycin and amoxicillin/clavulanate. Physicians may also use antipseudomonal therapy iv or by inhalation in cystic fibrosis.
- Treatment aimed at improving respiratory function is also required, including bronchodilators, physiotherapy and oxygen.

Prevention

- Good medical management of the airways disease and judicious use of antibiotics may prevent developing infection.
- Prophylactic antibiotics may have a role in patients with chronic lung disease.
- Vaccination against influenza is wise.

Acute bronchiolitis

Causative agent

- RSV in 75% of cases.
- Para-influenza, influenza, adeno- and rhinoviruses are the organisms responsible for the remainder.

Epidemiology

- These agents are a common cause of upper and lower respiratory tract infections during the winter months.
- The viruses are droplet spread.
- Bronchiolitis is a disease of children under the age of 2 years.
- Older children and adults will suffer prolonged coryza with RSV infection, but the elderly may develop bronchopneumonia. Immunity is short-lived and incomplete.

Incubation period

- Usually 2–8 days.

Clinical features

- After an initial prodromal period of coryza lasting 1–5 days, the child becomes more breathless, with a cough productive of copious mucoid sputum and developing respiratory distress. At this stage, the temperature is normal or only mildly raised.

- Examination reveals a breathless child using accessory muscles of inspiration. The chest is over-expanded and, on auscultation, fine inspiratory crackles and expiratory wheezes will be heard.
- The child remains ill for 1–5 days, recovering totally by 2 weeks.
- The disease may progress to bronchopneumonia and respiratory failure.

Differential diagnosis

- The disease can have features that may suggest bronchitis, bronchopneumonia or asthma.

Diagnosis

- The chest X-ray will show hyper-expanded lung fields with minor patchy shadowing.
- The virus may be isolated by nasopharyngeal aspiration. RSV may be seen by immunofluorescent staining and can be grown on tissue culture.

Treatment

- The mainstay of therapy is oxygen administration and physiotherapy.
- Nebulized ribavirin has been shown to improve the prognosis of severe infection.
- Antibiotics, steroids and bronchodilators are of no proven value.

Prevention

- Isolation of the index case may reduce intrafamilial spread.

Lung abscess and aspiration pneumonia

Causative agents

- *Streptococcus milleri*, and anaerobic cocci and bacilli, *Klebsiella pneumoniae*, *Staph. aureus*, *S. pyogenes* and *S. pneumoniae* – often polymicrobial.
- Rarely, septic emboli from tonsillitis due to *Fusobacterium necrophorum* ('necrobacillosis').

Epidemiology

● Anaerobic lung abscess and aspiration pneumonia arise after loss of consciousness in alcoholics, epileptics, drug addicts, head injury patients and postoperatively.
● Aerobic abscess occurs in severe primary pneumonias due to *Staph. aureus*, *Klebsiella pneumoniae* and *S. pneumoniae* in particular.
● Anaerobic infections are more likely in patients with carious teeth and gingivitis.
● Embolic abscesses will arise from distant sites of infection, e.g. staphylococcal endocarditis.

Incubation period

● 7–12 days after aspiration.

Clinical features

● Aerobic lung abscess occurs during acute pneumonia, as described previously (page 32).
● Anaerobic infections present with the slow development of low-grade fever, malaise and cough, producing copious amounts of sputum which is often foul-smelling.
● All infections can be complicated by empyema and lung damage. The aerobic infections may also progess to septicaemia. A mortality rate of 10–20% is seen depending on the cause.

Differential diagnosis

● Bronchitis, bronchopneumonia, bronchiectasis and other lobar pneumonias must be considered.
● TB, carcinoma of the bronchus and fungal infections also cause cavitation.

Diagnosis

● The chest X-ray will show lobar consolidation with single or multiple cavities when an abscess complicates acute pneumonia.
● Aspiration pneumonia will be most commonly seen in the posterior segment of the right or left upper lobes, or the apical segments of the lower lobes which are the most dependent in the horizontal patient.
● The organisms may be grown from sputum, blood or material aspirated directly from an abscess.

Treatment

- When aspiration pneumonia is suspected, therapy with parenteral benzylpenicillin 20–50 mg/kg, 6 hourly, with metronidazole 7 mg/kg, 8 hourly, should be given for 2–4 weeks. Chest physiotherapy is also helpful.
- Specific therapy of other organisms is as stated in the section on acute pneumonias (*see* page 33).
- Chest physiotherapy is unhelpful in other acute lobar pneumonias (non-aspiration).

Prevention

- Physiotherapy and postural drainage postoperatively may prevent such complications.

Pleural empyema

Causative agents

- *Staph. aureus.*
- *S. pneumoniae.*
- *S. pyogenes.*
- *Streptococcus milleri.*
- Anaerobes.
- In the immunocompromised, Gram-negative bacilli are important causes.

Epidemiology and pathophysiology

- The infection may follow pneumonia.
- The infection can also complicate trauma, haemothorax and pneumothorax, and be a super-infection of a previous pleural effusion.

Clinical features

- These include fever, chest pain, dyspnoea and weight loss. Fever in a person with a known pleural effusion should also raise suspicion.
- Physical examination reveals a dull percussion note and decreased breath sounds over the affected area.

Differential diagnosis

● Pleural effusion related to malignancy and TB should be excluded.

Diagnosis

● A plain chest X-ray will usually reveal the typical features of fluid with an upper meniscus and a level that changes with position, although some empyemas are loculated.
● CT scanning will delineate the collection of pus.
● The white blood cell count will be raised.
● The bacterium can be identified in aspirated fluid.

Treatment

● Treatment depends on a combination of surgical drainage and prolonged parenteral antibiotics appropriate to the organism (*see* acute pneumonias, page 33).

Tuberculosis

Causative agents

● *Mycobacterium tuberculosis.*
● *Mycobacterium bovis.*

Epidemiology and pathophysiology

● The disease occurs throughout the world, but in the UK manifest disease is confined mainly to defined groups: ethnic minorities, especially Asian, alcoholics, the immunocompromised, diabetics and the elderly.
● *Mycobacterium tuberculosis* is spread via respiratory droplets, *Mycobacterium bovis* from infected cow's milk.
● Both conditions are falling in incidence, especially infection with *Mycobacterium bovis* after it was virtually eradicated from British cattle. In 1990 in England and Wales 5282 cases were notified, including 290 deaths. An increase in the number of cases is predicted due to HIV infection.

Incubation period

● 6–14 weeks after first exposure; however, most cases are 'post primary', many years later.

Clinical features

- The disease is divided into primary and post-primary infections.
- Primary infection occurs in children and young adults after first exposure. A primary ('Ghon') focus occurs where the organism first infects tissue. Most commonly, this is detected in the lung with a confined granulomatous reaction peripherally in the middle lobe and an associated hilar lymphadenopathy. A primary focus may also occur in the pharynx with cervical adenopathy, or the intestine with mesenteric adenopathy. In 85–90% of cases, the lesion heals leaving minor fibrosis as the only manifestation. Primary infection is often asymptomatic.
- In a minority, the infection is not so confined and progression to massive mediastinal lymphadenopathy, tuberculous broncho-pneumonia, miliary TB and meningitis may occur.
- Post-primary TB is seen in older children and adults and arises either from reactivation of quiescent infection or re-infection.
- The most common manifestation in this group is with lung disease. Onset is slow with developing fever, weight loss, night sweats and cough productive of green or blood-stained sputum. Typically, several weeks elapse before diagnosis. Occasionally, an extensive bronchopneumonia with severe symptoms, including dyspnoea, can be seen.
- Other presentations include: fever and lymphadenopathy (usually cervical) in approximately 10% of Asian cases; miliary TB, with fever and profound weight loss progressing to meningitis and death if untreated; focal infection of kidney, genital tract, the meninges and other tissues can also be seen.
- Physical signs depend on the site of infection, but include weight loss and fever varying from 37–40°C. In early pulmonary TB, chest signs are absent or confined to localized inspiratory crackles. Signs of disease elsewhere are usually confined to the systemic effects, although bone pain, haematuria or microscopic pyuria, pelvic pain and infertility will indicate the infected site. TB meningitis can be a particularly difficult diagnosis presenting with fever and non-specific headache. Neck stiffness, photophobia, decreased consciousness and focal neurological signs are late signs.
- Erythema nodosum and erythema induratum, nodular eruptions on the front and back of the legs, respectively, are occasional associations with this infection.

Differential diagnosis

- This disease can be mimicked by a large number of diseases depending on the site.

Diagnosis

- It is important to be aware of TB as the possible cause of any febrile episode in the patient groups described above.
- Pulmonary TB is suggested by patchy shadowing that is usually localized and mostly confined to the lung apices. Cavitation is often present. Sputum staining with Ziehl–Nielsen or auramine stains and culture on Lowenstein–Jensen medium will confirm the diagnosis in the majority of cases. Bronchoscopy or early morning gastric lavage are helpful in sputum-negative cases.
- Tuberculin testing is of dubious value, because it merely reflects immunity. This investigation in the form of Mantoux, Heaf or tine (Rosenthal) tests, can be negative in primary infections, severe disease and the immunocompromised. It may be strongly positive in previously vaccinated patients who have been re-exposed but not re-infected. A positive test, indicated by induration after 72 hours of >10 mm following intradermal injection of 1 or 10 tuberculin units in 0.1 ml for the Mantoux test, is suggestive of active infection and warrants further investigation.
- The white blood count is usually normal but a raised erythrocyte sedimentation rate (ESR) and abnormal liver function tests may be detected.
- Confirmation of focal disease depends on isolation of the bacterium from affected tissue or secretions.
- In miliary TB the chest X-ray may reveal widespread 1–2-mm nodular opacities, but, in the presence of a normal chest X-ray, diagnosis is most commonly achieved by seeking granulomas or bacilli on liver biopsy or seeing organisms on marrow aspiration.
- TB meningitis is diagnosed by lumbar puncture, revealing a raised lymphocyte count and protein levels in the CSF, with a normal or low glucose and normal or high pressure. The organism will be seen on microscopy in only 30% of cases, although it is more frequently cultured.

Treatment

- The main drugs are rifampicin 10 mg/kg up to 600 mg, isoniazid 5 mg/kg up to 300 mg, pyrazinamide 20–35 mg/kg, ethambutol 15–25 mg/kg and streptomycin 20–40 mg/kg up to 2 g, all daily. These are usually given as an initial combination of 3 or 4 drugs for 2 months, with 2 drugs, usually rifampicin and isoniazid, continued for a further 4–7 months in pulmonary TB, and up to 22 more months for other sites of infection. Higher doses may be used in meningitis.

- These drugs have a wide range of side-effects, including fever (most drugs), hepatotoxicity (all except ethambutol), peripheral neuropathy (isoniazid), optic neuritis (ethambutol), red secretions and inhibition of the oral contraceptive pill (rifampicin).
- Drug resistance is found in imported strains of *Mycobacterium tuberculosis* and sensitivity testing should be carried out on cultured specimens.
- The use of steroid therapy is controversial.

Prevention

- All cases of TB should be notified to the medical officer of environmental health or CCDC, by telephone in cases of sputum–microscopy-positive cases.
- Contacts of infectious cases should be investigated by chest X-ray and tuberculin testing. A changing or suspicious chest X-ray, or changing tuberculin reaction, suggests exposure and may warrant therapy.
- Infectious cases are isolated until chemotherapy is felt to have rendered them of low risk (usually after 2 weeks).
- BCG vaccination is administered to Caucasian teenagers or to newborn infants in ethnic minorities in the UK. Its efficacy is still debatable.
- Chemoprophylalxis with isoniazid or rifampicin and isoniazid is sometimes given to people at high risk of developing infection, such as those whose tuberculin reaction has become strongly positive, especially children, or immunocompromised patients with a recent history of active TB.

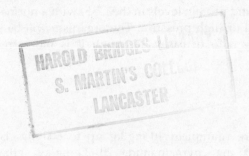

CHAPTER 5

Infections of the heart

CARDIAC infections are rare, except perhaps for the very mild transient myocarditis that accompanies a variety of viral diseases. This is fortunate in the light of the considerable morbidity and mortality associated with these infections. Although rheumatic fever now occurs infrequently, it has been included to emphasize its historical importance and to keep the possibility of this diagnosis in mind so that such patients can receive early recognition and optimal therapy.

Infective endocarditis

Causative agents

- Viridans streptococci (30–40%).
- *Enterococcus faecalis* (5–18%).
- Other streptococci (mainly *S. bovis*) (15–25%).
- *Staph. aureus* (10–27%).
- Coagulase-negative staphylococci (1–3%).
- Gram-negative bacilli in drug abusers and those with prosthetic heart valves (1–13%).
- Fungi (2–4%).
- *Coxiella burnetii* (1%).

Epidemiology and pathophysiology

- The disease is classified as acute when septicaemia leads to infection of a usually normal heart valve or as subacute when the heart valve, which was previously abnormal, is infected after minor bacteraemia.
- The more virulent organisms may cause acute endocarditis in drug addicts, patients with iv cannulae and others with pre-existing infection elsewhere.
- The subacute form is seen in patients who have congenital heart disease, valve damage due to rheumatic fever or prosthetic heart valves.
- Infection in those with prosthetic heart valves sometimes follows dentistry and minor surgery.

Incubation period

- Usually 2 weeks.

Clinical features

- Symptoms and signs can be very non-specific, and the diagnosis of this condition requires a high index of suspicion.
- The commonest symptoms are fever (95%), rigors (40%), malaise (40%), dyspnoea (40%), sweating, weight loss and anorexia (25%), neurological deficit (20%), and chest pain (15%).
- Physical signs are protean and can include fever (95%), heart murmur (85%), embolic phenomena (50%), splinter haemorrhages (15%), Osler's nodes (10–20%), finger-clubbing (10–50%), and spleno-megaly (20–50%).
- The usual presentation of subacute cases is of prolonged (>2 weeks) fever and malaise often in a patient who is known to have a heart-valve lesion, prosthetic valve or a congenital heart defect. In addition to the physical signs listed above, haematuria will usually be found on urine testing. A history of dental work or recent minor surgery is frequently obtained.
- The more fulminant cases present as high fever with appropriate physical signs as listed above. Congestive cardiac failure or cardio-genic shock may ensue.
- In untreated cases, the patient is at risk of valve destruction and cardiac failure, septic emboli leading to disseminated abscesses, infarcts, including stroke, and renal failure, leading to death.

Differential diagnosis

- This can be wide because the disease presents non-specifically in many cases.
- The vasculitic phenomena, such as splinter haemorrhage, may be found in a large number of patients who have infective or auto-immune disease.

Diagnosis

- The diagnosis should be considered in any patient in the known risk groups who presents with a fever lasting for more than a few days.
- Initial investigations will usually reveal a raised ESR, a high white blood cell count and blood (microscopic or macroscopic) in the urine. The blood urea is often raised.
- At least 3 blood cultures should be taken before empirical treatment is commenced.
- In culture-negative cases, consideration should be given to cultures for fungi and the more unusual bacteria, and antibody testing should be undertaken for 'atypical' organisms such as *Coxiella burnetii*.

- The chest X-ray, electrocardiogram (ECG) and echocardiogram will all give useful information.

Treatment

- When the diagnosis is highly likely, but before blood cultures become positive, empirical therapy with benzylpenicillin 50 mg/kg, every 4–6 hours, and gentamicin 1.7 mg/kg, every 8–12 hours, both iv, should be started. In drug addicts and others at risk of being infected by *Staph. aureus*, flucloxacillin 30–60 mg/kg, 6 hourly, may be added.
- Continuing therapy then depends on the antibiotic sensitivities of the isolated organism, but in culture-negative cases the above regimen may be continued.
- Cardiac surgery is often required, and should be considered in patients with developing evidence of cardiac dysfunction or indices of continuing infection despite adequate antibiotic therapy and a sensitive organism.

Prevention

- Patients who have a cardiac malformation, heart-valve damage or a prosthetic valve should receive antibiotic prophylaxis for dental and other minor surgical procedures. The prophylactic regimen is changed occasionally and, if in doubt, up to date advice should be sought. Recent recommendations include the following.

1 Dental surgery under local anaesthetic: amoxycillin 3 g 1 hour prior to the procedure, or erythromycin 1.5 g 1 hour before and 500 mg 6 hours after if the patient is allergic to penicillin. If the patient has had endocarditis previously, gentamicin is given with the amoxycillin as above.
2 Dental surgery under general anaesthetic: amoxycillin 3 g 4 hours before and 3 g as soon as possible after the procedure, or amoxycillin 1 g given im or iv at induction plus 500 mg orally 6 hours later, or amoxycillin 3 g plus probenecid 1 g 4 hours prior to surgery.
3 High-risk patients (i.e. those with a prosthetic valve or who have had previous endocarditis) should have amoxycillin 1 g given im or iv plus gentamicin 1.5 mg/kg at induction then oral amoxycillin 500 mg 6 hours later.
4 If patients are allergic to penicillin, then vancomycin 1 g given as a 60-minute iv infusion and gentamicin 1.5 mg/kg im or iv at induction.
5 Abdominal procedures: amoxycillin and gentamicin, or vancomycin with gentamicin, should be given as described above.

Myocarditis/pericarditis

Causative agents

- Enteroviruses, particularly Coxsackie B, are the commonest cause.
- A large number of other viruses, bacteria and fungi have been implicated.

Epidemiology

- The enteroviruses are common respiratory tract pathogens transmitted by droplet and faeco-oral spread, mainly in the summer and autumn.
- Any age-group may be affected.

Incubation period

- 5 days for the enteroviruses.

Clinical features

- Myocarditis varies from an asymptomatic disease detected incidentally to rapidly progressive heart failure.
- Specific features include tachycardia out of proportion to other symptoms, progressive cardiac failure or dysrhythmias.
- Examination reveals a normal or large heart beating fast or irregularly, and sometimes evidence of cardiac failure. There may be associated features of pericarditis.
- Pericarditis usually presents with central chest pain, which radiates to the shoulder and neck, exacerbated by deep breathing, swallowing and the supine position.
- A pericardial rub may be heard.
- There may be associated fever, 'flu-like illness or symptoms of an upper respiratory infection in both conditions.
- Myocarditis may progress to death from cardiac failure or cardiac arrest.
- Pericarditis usually resolves, but occasionally cardiac tamponade, with developing hypotension, can develop.

Differential diagnosis

- Mycocarditis may be difficult to distinguish from other forms of heart-muscle disease, including the cardiomyopathies, and hypertensive and ischaemic heart diseases (IHD).

- Pericarditis may be caused by a variety of non-infective processes, including post-myocardial infarction (MI), autoimmune diseases, malignancy, uraemia, drugs, sarcoidosis and hypothyroidism.
- Acute bacterial and tuberculous pericarditis are important to recognize.

Diagnosis

- In both cases, the chest X-ray may show cardiac silhouette enlargement. Additionally, myocarditis may be associated with features of pulmonary oedema.
- The echocardiogram and ECG will confirm the diagnosis.
- Enterovirus and other specific viral causes can be confirmed by serological means, or appropriate cultures, e.g. stool.
- In suspected bacterial or fungal pericarditis, pericardiocentesis may be required to both drain accumulating fluid and identity the organism.

Treatment

- In the majority of cases, therapy is aimed at relieving symptoms until recovery occurs naturally.
- Antimicrobial therapy is required in bacterial and fungal infections.
- Immunosuppression has occasionally been beneficial in severe enteroviral myocarditis.
- Surgery is necessary in exceptional cases to relieve the constrictive pericarditis that may ensue, and heart transplantation may be a last resort when severe damage to the heart muscle has occurred.

Prevention

- There is no potential for reducing the incidence of any of these conditions.

Rheumatic fever

Causative agent

- S. pyogenes (Lancefield Group A β-haemolytic streptococci).

Epidemiology

- This is most frequently a disease of children aged 6–15 years.
- The disease follows streptococcal tonsillitis/pharyngitis.

- The incidence is higher in lower socio-economic groups and among those living in crowded conditions.
- The incidence of rheumatic fever has been falling steadily this century, with an attack rate of approximately 0.5/100 000 population per year at present.

Incubation period

- 1–5 weeks after the streptococcal infection.

Clinical features

- Although the disease is a sequela of streptococcal infection, the mechanism is unknown.
- The syndrome is a collection of symptoms and signs that individually can have a variety of causes, but together suggest this single aetiology.
- Most usually an attack follows a symptomatic streptococcal infection and presents with fever and flitting arthritis of medium-sized joints, which may also be accompanied by carditis with developing heart murmurs.
- Other manifestations, such as the rash of erythema marginatum – large red circular lesions with a clear centre that change rapidly – and Sydenham's chorea are less frequent.
- The disease will eventually remit after approximately 12 weeks, leaving heart-valve damage in decreasing frequency of mitral, aortic, and tricuspid or pulmonary valves in approximately 50% of cases.
- Death is unusual in the acute attack, but severe myocarditis can be fatal.
- Rheumatic fever may recur after subsequent streptococcal infections.

Differential diagnosis

- The individual symptoms can be similar to a variety of diseases, but the more features present, the greater the likelihood of rheumatic fever.

Diagnosis

- Diagnosis is formalized in the Jones criteria. It depends on the following.

1 Evidence of recent streptococcal infection in a raised antistreptolysin O (ASO) or other streptococcal antibody titre, a positive culture of *S. pyogenes*, or definite scarlet fever.

2 Two major, or one major and two minor criteria, being present. (*See* Table 5.1)

Table 5.1 The Jones criteria used in the diagnosis of rheumatic fever

Major criteria
- Flitting polyarthritis
- Carditis
- Sydenham's chorea
- Erythema marginatum
- Subcutaneous nodules

Minor criteria
- Past rheumatic fever
- Arthralgia
- Fever
- Acute-phase reactants (raised ESR, C reactive protein (CRP), white blood cell count, etc.)
- Prolonged P–R interval on ECG

Treatment
- Aspirin or other non-steroidal anti-inflammatory drugs (NSAIDs) are of benefit for arthritis and arthralgia.
- Penicillin is also usually given to eradicate any persisting streptococci.
- The role of steroids is controversial, but despite many advocates it is of no definite value.
- Treatment may have to be continued for many weeks.

Prevention
- Although the falling incidence of rheumatic fever has coincided with increasing use of antibiotics, there is no clear evidence that the relationship is causal. As many cases of rheumatic fever occur after streptococcal infections that do not require antibiotic therapy, the liberal use of these agents is unlikely to reduce the attack rate.
- When a patient has suffered from proven rheumatic fever, penicillin prophylaxis is given for at least 5 years and until the age of 20 years. Prophylaxis can be given as monthly im injections of benzathine penicillin 0.6–1.2 M units or twice daily oral penicillin V 4 mg/kg.

CHAPTER 6

Gastrointestinal infection and food poisoning

THIS group of infections includes some of the commonest causes of serious infection. There are many misconceptions about the management of the diarrhoeal diseases. Most of these infections are self-limiting, and antibiotics have little or no place in their therapy. Important exceptions are their use in giardiasis, and very early on in campylobacter infection, non-sonnei shigella dysentery and pseudo-membranous colitis. Often, antidiarrhoea drugs cause problems through their disposition to enhance tissue invasion by the bacteria, and also because of the patient's reliance on these agents, in contrast to bowel-rest and rehydration which are more important.

Although therapy is rarely changed on the basis of aetiological diagnosis, such a diagnosis is still necessary to enable public health measures, such as the investigation of food outlets, to be instituted by the local environmental health officers where appropriate. There is therefore a need for notification of relevant infections, particularly those due to *Salmonella* sp., as soon as possible (*see* Disease notification, page 219).

Not all gastrointestinal infections are caused by agents transmitted by food and water. An addition to the list of newly recognized infectious agents is *Helicobacter pylori*, now a confirmed cause of gastritis which is therefore included in this chapter.

Helicobacter pylori-related gastritis and peptic ulcer disease

Causative agent

- *Helicobacter pylori*, a Gram-negative bacillus (in 50% or more of cases).

Epidemiology

- Little is known at present about the transmission of this organism although person-to-person spread is likely.

Incubation period

- Unknown, but may be short.

Clinical features

- After acute experimental infection, nausea, vomiting and epigastric pain lasting several days occurs.
- Chronic infection is related to some cases of non-ulcer dyspepsia and peptic ulceration.

Differential diagnosis

- Acute infection must be distinguished from toxin-related vomiting and winter vomiting disease.
- Chronic infection is similar to idiopathic gastritis and peptic ulceration.

Diagnosis

- Diagnosis is confirmed by finding urease activity on gastric biopsy. The organism may also be grown or visualized from biopsy specimens.
- A radiolabelled ^{14}C-urea breath test can be used as a non-invasive investigation.

Treatment

- Bismuth salts for 4 weeks, with amoxycillin or metronidazole for 2 weeks, are most likely to be effective for chronic gastritis.
- Peptic ulcer disease may also require H_2-antagonists or omeprazole.

Prevention

- There is no known measure at present.

Viral gastroenteritis

Causative agents

- Rotavirus.
- Calicivirus, Norwalk agent, Astrovirus and other small round structured viruses (SRSVs).
- Adenovirus.

Epidemiology

- The viruses can be droplet or faeco-oral spread (rotavirus, adenovirus, the SRSVs involved in winter vomiting disease, Norwalk agent) or food-borne (some SRSVs).

- Rotavirus infection is primarily a disease of children, occurring most commonly in the winter months, although any age-group can be affected.
- The other viruses can infect people of any age, again with a winter preponderance.
- Food-borne outbreaks of infection due to SRSVs have been seen.

Incubation period

- Usually 2–4 days.

Clinical features

- These agents all cause diarrhoea which can be profuse and watery, and fever (37.5–39°C) which rarely lasts more than 1 week. There may be associated vomiting.
- In rotavirus and adenovirus infections particularly, there may be associated symptoms of upper respiratory tract infection and a transient maculopapular rash.
- The major complications include dehydration and secondary lactase deficiency in infants.
- Winter vomiting disease, a short-lived (<24 hours) episode of severe vomiting is due to SRSVs, including Norwalk agent.

Differential diagnosis

- The more severe cases can be similar to bacterial gastroenteritis.
- Winter vomiting disease causes symptoms that are almost identical with those of toxin-induced vomiting.

Diagnosis

- Diagnosis can be confirmed by electron microscopy of the stool or vomitus.

Treatment

- Oral or iv hydration is the only therapy usually required.
- A lactose or other disaccharide-free diet is occasionally required for infants who are intolerant of these sugars. This may be necessary for up to 3 months.

Salmonella gastroenteritis

Causative agents

- There are over 2000 serotypes of salmonella, the most commonly isolated in human disease being *Salmonella enteritidis* and *Salmonella typhimurium*. Salmonellae are Gram-negative bacilli.

Epidemiology

- Salmonellae infect a wide range of animals and may cause human disease when ingested with food.
- The infectious dose is large ($>10^5$ organisms), and an amplification stage is normally required for infection. This can occur when contaminated food is allowed to stand at room temperature for several hours. Rapid multiplication of the organism under these conditions provides bacterial levels adequate for infection unless the food is effectively cooked.
- Common food sources include poultry and other meats. *Salmonella enteritidis* phage type 4 is now the most frequently isolated salmonella and relates to the increasing infection of chickens, and in particular the abililty of this organism to infect the inside of eggs.
- Infection can be acquired from other sources including direct person-to-person contact, as sometimes seen in large institutional outbreaks, and from puppies and kittens.
- There are approximately 30 000 cases reported each year in England and Wales.
- Large outbreaks involving food served at functions are regularly detected.

Incubation period

- 12–72 hours; occasionally up to 7 days.

Clinical features

- Symptoms vary from mild or asymptomatic to severe gastroenteritis.
- The illness may be preceded by a short prodromal illness of fever, headache and myalgia, followed by the sudden onset of profuse vomiting and watery malodorous diarrhoea. The temperature may be as high as 40°C. Symptoms last for 1–7 days.
- Additional features may include colicky abdominal pain or blood and mucus in the stool.

- Dehydration may complicate severe diarrhoea, which in turn occasionally results in hypotension and renal failure.
- Other complications include bacteraemia and metastatic infection, such as osteomyelitis and soft tissue abscess; salmonella osteomyelitis is particularly common in the setting of sickle-cell anaemia.
- Post-diarrhoeal arthritis can occur.

Differential diagnosis

- This disease can be similar to the illnesses caused by *Shigella*, *Campylobacter*, *Yersinia*, pathogenic *Escherichia coli* and *Entamoeba histolytica*.

Diagnosis

- The organism will be found on culture of the stool.
- It is important to perform blood cultures in the debilitated patient and in those suffering prolonged disease in order to detect bacteraemia.
- The white blood cell count is usually normal or low, and the blood urea may be raised.

Treatment

- Therapy is primarily aimed at the prevention of dehydration with oral rehydration mixtures, although iv fluids are occasionally required.
- Antidiarrhoeal agents have little part to play, although analgesics may be required.
- Antibiotic therapy with chloramphenicol 10 mg/kg, 6 hourly, or ciprofloxacin 10 mg/kg, 12 hourly, both given orally for at least 5 days is required for detected bacteraemia, when the clinical situation suggests a severe bacteraemic illness or in the elderly and immuno-compromised with severe prolonged disease.
- In the rare case of chronic salmonella carriage, ciprofloxacin given for 2 weeks can effectively eradicate this state.

Prevention

- Most cases will be prevented by good food hygiene. In particular, food should be thoroughly cooked to ensure high temperatures in the centre. Eggs should be cooked until solid.
- Infected food handlers should be excluded from work until a minimum of six consecutive negative stool samples have been obtained. This is usually carried out by the local environmental health department. Other people can return to work on cessation of diarrhoea.

- There is a policy of detection and slaughter of poultry flocks infected with *Salmonella enteritidis* phage type 4 in the UK.
- The disease is notifiable and in cases of suspected outbreaks the responsible authorities should be notified by telephone.

Campylobacter gastroenteritis

Causative agents

- *Campylobacter jejuni* and *Campylobacter coli*, comma-shaped Gram-negative bacilli.

Incubation period

- 1–7 days, usually 2–4 days.

Epidemiology

- Campylobacter are commonly found in the intestine of many animals including dogs, sheep and especially poultry.
- It can be contracted from water, food, especially poorly cooked chicken, and unpasteurized milk. Person-to-person transmission is unusual. Domestic animals, especially cats and dogs, may also transmit to humans.
- Unlike salmonellae, campylobacter do not multiply in food and the potential for epidemics is reduced.
- It is second only to salmonella as a cause of bacterial food poisoning.

Clinical features

- Fever (up to 40°C), myalgia and abdominal pain often precede the diarrhoea.
- Stool volumes are large, in contrast to the small stool of shigella infections, watery and offensive and often contain blood and mucus.
- Vomiting is not usually a feature in adults, but is more commonly seen in children.
- A constant central abdominal plain associated also with a colicky abdominal pain temporarily relieved by defaecation is more characteristic of campylobacter infection than other similar illnesses.
- In 10% of cases, the course is prolonged (> 7 days) or relapsing.
- Complications include dehydration, toxic dilatation of the colon and post-diarrhoeal arthritis.

Differential diagnosis

- As for salmonella gastroenteritis.

Diagnosis

- The characteristic severe pain suggests the cause.
- It can be isolated from stool culture, although selective media, CO_2 enrichment, low O_2 and high temperatures (43°C) are required.

Treatment

- Fluid replacement is most important.
- Antidiarrhoeal agents may precipitate toxic dilatation of the colon.
- Analgesics are frequently required.
- Erythromycin or ciprofloxacin will reduce the disease duration and severity if given early, preferably in the first 48 hours.

Prevention

- Food hygiene and thorough cooking will reduce the incidence of infection.
- Antibiotic prophylaxis, while effective, is not recommended.

Bacillary dysentery (Shigella)

Causative agents

- *Shigella dysenteriae, Shigella flexneri, Shigella boydii.*

Epidemiology and pathophysiology

- The source of infection is usually the faeces of an infected patient or carrier.
- Infection spreads where hygiene is poor. Outbreaks are common in nurseries, primary schools and mental institutions.
- Some immunity is established as a result of an attack.
- 3603 reported cases of dysentery in England and Wales in 1987 including 3 deaths. 2805 cases in 1990. Increased incidence in the winter months.

Incubation period

- 2–4 days.

Clinical features

- Abrupt onset of fever, headache, colicky abdominal pain and vomiting, which does not persist.
- Diarrhoea, which may be severe and often contains blood and mucus.
- Febrile convulsions may occur in children and can be accompanied by tenesmus.
- Complications include haemorrhage from the bowel and ulcers which may lead to fibrosis and stenosis; arthritis; iritis.

Differential diagnosis

- Amoebic dysentery (see page 158) in travellers.
- In babies, intussusception should be suspected and may be difficult to distinguish clinically because of redcurrant stool appearance.
- In adults ulcerative colitis and Crohn's disease.
- In the elderly, ischaemic colitis, diverticulitis and carcinoma.

Diagnosis

- Isolation of the organism from stool; rectal swabs are not reliable.

Treatment

- Maintain fluid balance.
- For treatment of severe cases use ciprofloxacin 10 mg/kg twice a day for 5 days.

Prevention

- Strict hygiene particularly with food.
- Food handlers should usually be excluded from their work until stool cultures are negative.

Yersinia enteritis

Causative agents

- *Yersinia enterocolitica* and *Yersinia pseudotuberculosis*, Gram-negative bacilli.

Epidemiology

- These agents are via infected food (including unpasteurized milk) or by person-to-person spread.
- It is rarely seen in the UK.

Incubation period

- 3–7 days.

Clinical features

- The infection may present as an acute gastroenteritis similar to salmonella infection or dysentery, and is seen mostly in children.
- Older patients may present with fever and right iliac fossa pain, with little or no diarrhoea.
- 10–30% of adults develop a reactive medium-joint polyarthritis up to 1 month later.
- Erythema nodosum, *Yersinia enterocolitcia* septicaemia and mesenteric adenitis can also be seen.

Differential diagnosis

- The acute gastroenteritis is similar to that caused by other bacterial pathogens.
- The sub-acute form may mimic Crohn's disease and other focal intra-abdominal inflammatory conditions.

Diagnosis

- Diagnosis is made by isolation of the organism from faeces, mesenteric lymph nodes, peritoneal fluid or blood culture.
- A rising agglutination antibody titre in serum is also diagnostic.

Treatment

- Most cases are mild and self-limiting.
- Chronic infection will respond to a variety of antibiotics, including aminoglycosides, co-trimoxozale, tetracycline, ampicillin or a third-generation cephalosporin.

Prevention

- Personal and food hygiene.
- Pasteurization of milk.

Pathogenic Escherichia coli-related diarrhoea

Causative agents

- *E. coli*, a Gram-negative bacillus. Different serotypes have been linked to the various diarrhoeal syndromes.

Epidemiology

- Enterotoxigenic *E. coli* (ETEC) is discussed in Chapter 14 (page 158).
- Enteropathogenic *E. coli* (EPEC) strains cause illness mainly in infants. Their mode of acquisition in sporadic cases is not understood although infant-to-infant spread, often via their carers, is seen in institutional outbreaks. The incidence of this infection is falling in the UK.
- Entero-invasive (EIEC) strains are most likely spread by direct person-to-person or faeco-oral contact.
- Entero-haemorrhagic *E. coli*, otherwise known as vero-toxin producing *E. coli* (VTEC), are food-borne. The majority of infections are caused by the sorbitol non-fermenting 0157 serotype. Sporadic causes are seen in the UK, with occasional small epidemics, whereas in Canada this organism is one of the commonest causes of food poisoning.

Incubation period

- 1–2 days for ETEC.
- 1–3 days for EPEC, EIEC and VTEC.

Clinical features

- EPEC causes diarrhoea mainly in infants under the age of 4 months. Large outbreaks have been seen in nurseries.
- There is often a prodromal illness of up to 6 days where the infant is irritable and lethargic. This is followed by watery diarrhoea with little fever or vomiting. Diarrhoea can persist for up to 2 weeks during which period severe dehydration can be seen. Complications include disaccharide intolerance, venous thrombosis, pneumonia, peritonitis and septicaemia.

- EIEC causes a disease that is identical in manifestations to shigella dysentry with blood-stained diarrhoea and fever lasting for up to 2 weeks. It is uncommon and seen sporadically in all age-groups. Food transmission associated with cheese has been seen on one occasion.
- The diarrhoea caused by VTEC is also usually haemorrhagic, although fever is usually mild or absent. The illness can last several weeks and occasional cases of chronic diarrhoea, similar to inflammatory bowel disease, have been seen. Up to 90% of haemolytic-uraemic syndrome cases are related to this infection.

Differential diagnosis

- EPEC is similar to severe rotavirus- and adenovirus-related gastroenteritis.
- EIEC or VTEC must be distinguished from dysentery, invasive salmonella and campylobacter infections, idiopathic inflammatory bowel disease and pseudomembranous colitis.

Diagnosis

- Diagnosis is established by stool culture. The microbiologist should be requested to look specifically for the pathogenic *E. coli* as the stool always contains non-pathogenic serotypes.

Treatment

- Rehydration is the mainstay of therapy, although EPEC diarrhoea may be treated with non-absorbable antibiotics.
- Systemic antibiotics are occasionally required in severe EPEC infections.
- There is conflicting evidence on antibiotic therapy for VTEC-related illness; in some reports, a worse prognosis has been reported after such treatment.

Prevention

- EPEC and EIEC will continue to become less common as long as good standards of hygiene, such as handwashing, are maintained.
- VTEC-related infection can be controlled only by adequate cooking of contaminated food.

Pseudomembranous and post-antibiotic colitis

Causative agents

● *Clostridium difficile*, an anaerobic Gram-positive bacillus.

Epidemiology

● Some patients taking antibiotics, notably clindamycin, lincomycin, ampicillin and amoxycillin, may eventually develop this syndrome.
● Recent abdominal surgery also predisposes the patient to this agent with devastating effects.
● Middle-aged and elderly patients and those with mechanical abnormalities of the bowel are most at risk.
● The organism can be spread from person to person and by the faeco-oral route. Hospital outbreaks can occur.

Incubation period

● Symptoms usually commence within 10 days of starting antibiotic treatment, although they may take up to 3 weeks to appear.

Clinical features

● Symptoms often begin usually after a course of broad-spectrum antibiotics, with profuse, watery mucoid stool, often containing blood, fever (up to 40°C) and abdominal pain.
● Occasionally abdominal distension may develop.
● Complications include electrolyte disturbance, hypo-albuminaemia, toxic megacolon or perforation of the large bowel.

Differential diagnosis

● This includes dysentery, inflammatory bowel disease, infection pathogenic with *E. coli* and severe salmonella or campylobacter infections.

Diagnosis

● Toxin is demonstrable in the faeces by immunofluorescent or tissue culture methods.
● Isolation of the organism in the faeces is not diagnostic because it may be a commensal.

- The diagnosis should be suspected in patients who have received antibiotics within a month of the onset of diarrhoea.
- Sigmoidoscopy often reveals a congested rectal mucosa with overlying grey–white plaques of pseudomembrane, but the latter is not invariable.

Treatment

- Stop broad-spectrum antibiotics.
- Oral vancomycin 3–7 mg/kg, 6 hourly, for 10 days is usually effective.
- Oral metronidazole 6 mg/kg, 8 hourly, for 10 days is a suitable alternative.

Prevention

- Good hygiene.
- Isolation of affected patients.
- Restrictive use of antibiotics.

Giardiasis

Causative agent

- *Giardia lamblia*, a protozoan.

Epidemiology

- It can be spread from one infected person to another via the faeco-oral route, particularly in pre-school children and nursery outbreaks.
- Waterborne spread is important, and epidemics in North America (Aspen, Colorado) and the Soviet Union (Leningrad) have been via this route.
- Children are most commonly infected in the UK, although adults may be affected when they acquire the disease abroad.
- 5311 cases were reported in England, Wales, Northern Ireland, Eire, Channel Islands and Isle of Man in 1987.

Incubation period

- 2 weeks.

Clinical features

- The illness has an acute onset with offensive, watery diarrhoea, profuse flatulence and abdominal distension. Symptoms may persist for 6 weeks or more.
- Fever is uncommon.
- Disease in children may cause failure to thrive.
- A secondary lactose intolerance may develop.

Differential diagnosis

- Mild disease can be similar to other non-haemorrhagic diarrhoeas.
- Chronic disease must be distinguished from other causes of malabsorption such as coeliac disease.

Diagnosis

- Diagnosis is by microscopic identification of cysts in fresh faeces or trophozoites in duodenal aspirate. The identification rate is low, and at least 3 stool samples should be examined.

Treatment

- Metronidazole 30 mg/kg daily for 3 days, or tinidazole 30 mg/kg as a single dose, is usually effective.

Prevention

- Good personal hygiene.
- Hygienic sewage disposal.
- Water purification for travellers.

Cryptosporidiosis

Causative agent

- *Cryptosporidium parvum*, a protozoan.

Epidemiology

- This organism commonly affects domestic and farm animals, and most cases arise from water contamination, although person-to-person spread can occur.
- It mainly affects children, the immunocompromised and travellers.

- Infection is most frequent in spring and autumn.
- Mild disease is common, accounting for approximately 1% of gastroenteritis.
- 9000 cases were reported to the Public Health Laboratory in 1989.

Incubation period

- About 2–14 days.

Clinical features

- Symptoms are usually mild, although they may be incapacitating in the immunocompromised.
- Diarrhoea is often watery and offensive, with many episodes in a day. Up to 17 litres of diarrhoea in a day have been reported; mucus or slime may occur but rarely blood. It lasts from 2 days to 3 weeks, averaging 6 days in the immunocompetent. Constipation alternating with diarrhoea may occur during convalescence. The diarrhoea is often chronic in AIDS patients.
- Vomiting, abdominal pain and weight loss may also be seen.
- Anorexia, fever, lethargy, nausea, headache, listlessness and arthritis can occur in immunocompromised (including pregnant) patients.
- A syndrome of right upper quadrant pain and a raised alkaline phosphatase, due to sclerosing cholangitis, has been attributed to cryptosporidia and cytomegalovirus (CMV) infection in AIDS.

Differential diagnosis

- Viral, mild bacterial and giardia-related gastroenteritis may present in a similar fashion.

Diagnosis

- Diagnosis is made after the examination of the faeces for oocysts. Oocysts may be excreted for several weeks after the diarrhoea has stopped.
- Rectal biopsy may be necessary.

Treatment

- Palliation with adequate fluids to prevent dehydration.
- Antibiotics are of no proven value and chronic cases in AIDS require therapy with antidiarrhoeal drugs.

Prevention

- Adequate filtration of water supplies will reduce the incidence.

Diseases due to food-borne bacterial toxins

Causative agents

- *Staph. aureus.*
- *Clostridium perfringens.*
- *Bacillus cereus.*
- *Clostridium botulinum.*

Epidemiology

- These organisms cause disease after multiplying and producing a toxin in food or after ensuing gut infection.
- *Staph. aureus* contaminates food, usually cold meats or dairy products, via a food handler with a staphylococcal infection or nasal carriage. The toxin is heat-labile and infection depends on lack of, or inadequate, cooking of the food.
- *Clostridium perfringens* also infects meat, fish and milk products, and is a ubiquitous soil organism whose spores contaminate the food. It can be destroyed by adequate cooking.
- *Bacillus cereus* was first recognized in poorly cooked fried rice. Other cereals, meat and milk products can be contaminated. The organism can produce two toxins: one heat-labile, the other heat-stable.
- *Clostridium botulinum* is strictly anaerobic and disease occurs when contaminated food is canned or bottled and the food incompletely sterilized. It is rare.
- 20 363 cases reported in England and Wales in 1987.

Incubation period

- *Staph. aureus* and short-incubation *Bacillus cereus*-related: 1–6 hours.
- Long-incubation *Bacillus cereus* and *Clostridium perfringens* infection: 8–16 hours.
- *Clostridium botulinum*: 12 hours to 8 days.

Clinical features

- Toxin disease due to *Staph. aureus* and *Bacillus cereus* presents with profound nausea and vomiting lasting 1–12 hours. Mild diarrhoea and low-grade fever may also be seen.

- *Clostridium perfringens* and long incubation-period *Bacillus cereus* disease cause watery diarrhoea lasting less than 24 hours. Nausea is common, although vomiting and fever are less common.
- Botulism, due to the toxin of *Clostridium botulinum* can begin with lethargy, nausea and vomiting, and dry mouth. Sooner or later neurological dysfunction is seen with diplopia and other cranial nerve palsies. Generalized motor and autonomic nerve paralysis occurs, leading to weakness, respiratory distress and postural hypertension. There is a high mortality (approximately 25%) proportional to the amount of weakness, which is inversely proportional to the incubation period.

Differential diagnosis

- Acute vomiting can be caused by winter vomiting disease, acute gastritis due to *Helicobacter pylori*, and ingestion of chemical poisons. Vomiting can also be the symptom of many severe systemic diseases.
- Watery diarrhoea without fever can also be caused by giardiasis, cryptosporidiosis and other less common intestinal protozoa. Viral and, less commonly, bacterial gastroenteritis may be short-lived.
- Botulism may be mistaken for Guillain–Barré syndrome, myasthenia gravis, poliomyelitis and poisoning due to organophosphorus compounds.

Diagnosis

- The diagnosis of toxin-related vomiting and diarrhoea is clinical, although the toxin can be found in the food source or vomitus.
- The diagnosis of botulism is mainly clinical, although the normal CSF in this condition distinguishes it from many other causes.
- Electromyography may show typical changes.
- The diagnosis is confirmed by finding botulinum toxin in the serum, or the toxin or organism in vomitus, stool or food source.

Treatment

- Vomiting and diarrhoea settle quickly, and require only fluid replacement.
- Botulism is treated by the use of polyvalent equine antitoxin with specificity against all known toxins (A–G). This is given parenterally and may be repeated after 2–4 hours. Availability is through the local public health laboratory.
- Therapy is otherwise supportive and usually requires intensive care with ventilatory support for the time (weeks or months) that paralysis may persist.

Prevention

- In each case, the illness will be avoided by good food hygiene and adequate refrigeration.
- Food handlers with overt staphylococcal lesions should be debarred until the lesions heal.

Table 6.1 A summary of gastrointestinal symptoms and their causative agents

Vomiting alone
- *Helicobacter pylori*
- SRSVs (winter vomiting disease)
- Toxins of *Staph. aureus* and *Bacillus cereus*

Watery diarrhoea without fever
- *Giardia lamblia*
- *Cryptosporidum parvum*
- *Bacillus cereus*
- *Clostridium perfringens* (rarely cholera)
(*NB:* in viral gastroenteritis the fever is often mild)

Watery diarrhoea and vomiting with fever
- *Salmonella* sp.
- *Campylobacter* sp.
- *Shigella sonnei*
- *E. coli* (EPEC)
- *Yersinia* sp.
- Viruses

Blood-stained diarrhoea
- *Salmonella* sp.
- *Campylobacter* sp.
- *Shigella* sp.
- *Clostridium difficile*
- *E. coli* (EIEC and VTEC)

CHAPTER 7

Infections of the liver and biliary system

ALTHOUGH hepatitis is a description of symptoms and signs that include jaundice, it is not in itself a diagnosis. In remembering this, the doctor will avoid the potential hazards of missing such serious but treatable conditions as cholangitis, leptospirosis and haemolytic anaemia. The correct aetiological diagnosis can be achieved first by avoiding a diagnosis of viral hepatitis in the patient over 40 years of age unless there is compelling evidence to the contrary. A diagnosis of obstructive biliary disease, caused by gallstones or malignancy, would be more likely. Second, the only viral hepatitis in which fever commonly persists after the first 2 days of jaundice is that due to EBV. Otherwise cholangitis, leptospirosis and, importantly, malaria and typhoid in the returned traveller should be given serious consideration. It is a sad fact that in infectious disease practice, more harm has been caused by the mis-diagnosis of the jaundiced patient than almost any other condition.

When a diagnosis of viral hepatitis is confirmed, the doctor's work has only begun. The proper use of preventive measures in contacts and the new potentials for therapy in severe or chronic disease mean that a great deal can be done to ameliorate the effects of these frequently devastating illnesses.

Hepatitis A

Causative agents

- Hepatitis A virus, a picornavirus.

Epidemiology

- It is spread by the faeco-oral route, including food (especially shell-fish), water contaminated by sewage and close personal contact.
- In developed countries, infection is mainly seen in children or young adults, although older people are not entirely immune.
- In developing countries, the virus is most often transmitted in childhood.
- Epidemics can occur in closed communities and institutions. Approximately 3000 cases per year are reported in the UK.

Incubation period

● 10–50 days.

Clinical features

● In children, the infection is usually asymptomatic and anicteric.
● Symptomatic disease commences with fever, myalgia, nausea, epigastric discomfort and a distaste for cigarettes. Arthritis and rash may also be seen. This prodromal illness lasts for 1–14 days.
● After the prodromal phase, the symptoms mainly subside as jaundice appears, accompanied by pale stools and dark urine. Fever is unusual in the icteric phase, whilst nausea and epigastric discomfort may persist. Jaundice disappears after 1–14 weeks.
● Complications include fulminant hepatic failure in <1% of cases, (presenting as increasing hepatic encephalopathy), and cholestatic hepatitis (where deep jaundice and severe itching may last several months). Chronic disease is unknown although relapses do occur.
● Examination in the prodromal phase will reveal no diagnostic features, whereas in the icteric period an enlarged, tender liver is usually felt, sometimes in association with splenomegaly (approximately 20%).

Differential diagnosis

● Other viral hepatitides.
● EBV-related hepatitis.
● Alcoholic and drug-induced hepatitis.
● Leptospirosis.
● Biliary tract obstruction.
● Haemolytic jaundice.

Diagnosis

● Liver function tests (LFT) show the characteristic hepatocullar pattern, i.e. raised bilirubin, aspartate aminotransferases (often >1000 iu/l) and a moderately raised alkaline phosphatase of up to twice the upper limit of normal. In the cholestatic variant, the alkaline phosphatase may be higher.
● Bile will be found in the urine.
● The hepatitis A virus IgM antibody test in serum will be positive.
● Hepatitis A is unlikely when fever persists after the first few days of jaundice.

Treatment

- Most patients feel better after 1–2 weeks of jaundice, although full recovery may take much longer. There is conflicting evidence on the merits of rest in the early phase. Some clinicians insist on bedrest until there is no bilirubinuria, whereas others maintain that patients can mobilize themselves as they feel able, as long as the amino-transferase levels are falling.
- Cholestatic hepatitis A will improve after a short course of steroids (prednisolone 0.6 mg/kg daily for 5 days).

Prevention

- Human normal immunoglobulin may prevent spread if given soon after contact with the index case, and in foreign travellers.
- Food hygiene is also important.

Hepatitis B

Causative agent

- Hepatitis B virus, an hepadnavirus.

Epidemiology

- In developed countries, hepatitis B is mainly a disease of adults, particularly male homosexuals, iv drug abusers, haemophiliacs, dialysis patients, those in institutions for the mentally retarded and, rarely post-transfusion – so-called 'horizontal transmission'. This is caused by contamination with blood or other body fluids.
- In ethnic minorities, particularly of South East Asian origin, it is commonly transmitted from infected mother to newborn child – the 'vertical' route. Infection in infants and pre-school children accounts for the majority of the world's 300 million infected individuals who for the most part live in South East Asia.
- There are at present approximately 500 new cases notified each year in England and Wales, and approximately 50 000 carriers.
- Up to 40% of notified cases of hepatitis B have no identifiable risk factor for infection.
- This infection is significantly associated with primary liver cancer, particularly in developing countries.

Incubation period

- 40–160 days.

Clinical features

- Asymptomatic, anicteric infection is common, particularly in the immunocompromised, such as HIV-infected individuals. Such episodes are more likely to proceed to chronic disease.
- Symptomatic disease is similar to that of acute hepatitis A virus infection, although it is more likely to be severe.
- Arthritis and the rash of angio-oedema are more common in hapatitis B virus infection.
- Other complications include glomerulonephritis, polyarteritis nodosum and aplastic anaemia.
- Most patients recover in 1–12 weeks, although approximately 1% follow a fulminant course with a mortality rate of about 40%. Chronic disease, defined as infection lasting for more than 6 months, occurs in about 10% of infected patients; this is more common in the immunocompromised.
- Chronic disease, particularly when associated with high aminotransferase levels and chronic active hepatitis on liver biopsy histology, can lead to cirrhosis in 10% of horizontally acquired and 50% of vertically and childhood infected cases. There is also a high (10%) risk of liver cancer in patients with cirrhosis.

Differential diagnosis

- *See* hepatitis A (page 71).
- In severe hepatitis B virus infection consider co-infection with delta virus (hepatitis D virus).

Diagnosis

- Hepatitis in those groups 'at risk' should raise the suspicion of hepatitis B virus infection.
- There are several serological markers of infection, namely surface antigen (HBsAg) and its antibody (anti-HBs), 'e' antigen (HBeAg) and antibody (anti-HBe) and anticore antibody (anti-HBc, IgG or IgM). The pattern of these markers indicates the stage of infection and infectivity as follows.

IgM anti-core: present in acute infection or, occasionally, in relapse of chronic infection.
HBsAg: present in acute or chronic infection. The serum may contain large amounts of excess HBsAg.
Anti-HBs: found in those who have suffered past infection or after immunization.

HBeAG: indicates active infection either acute or chronic, and is a marker of infectivity.

Anti-HBe: detected in recovered infection or chronic carriers, mainly of low infectivity; there are exceptions to this rule of infectivity in ethnic minorities.

Treatment

● Acute hepatitis B virus infection is managed as acute hepatitis A infection.
● Fulminant viral infection may require management in intensive care and, occasionally, liver transplantation.
● In a significant proportion of patients, chronic hepatitis B virus infection can be eradicated by antiviral agents, such as alpha-interferon and vidaribine-5'-monophosphate.

Prevention

● Infants born to HBsAg-positive mothers should receive active (HBsAg) and passive (anti-HBs) immunization.
● Immunization with these agents should also be offered to medical workers after needlestick injury or other contamination with infected material, or others at risk e.g. sexual contacts of known cases.
● Active immunization with the plasma-derived or newer recombinant vaccine should be offered to individuals at risk, such as health-care workers.

Hepatitis C (parenteral non-A non-B hepatitis)

Causative agent

● Hepatitis C virus, as yet an unclassified ribonucleic acid (RNA) virus.
● There may be other non-A non-B viruses.

Epidemiology

● This agent has recently been recognized as the major cause of acute and chronic hepatitis following blood and blood product transfusion. It is paticularly common in iv drug abusers and haemophiliacs.
● In the UK, there are an estimated 50 000 antibody-positive individuals.

- This agent has been linked to cirrhosis, particularly the 'cryptogenic' type, and liver cancer.
- 50% of antibody-positive individuals have *not* received transfusions; other routes of infection have not been defined as yet.

Incubation period

- 14–168 days.

Clinical features

- Acute hepatitis is normally mild with only 25% of cases being icteric, and other symptoms are rarely significant.
- Fulminant hepatitis, with a high mortality, is a rare complication.
- Up to 75% of infections become chronic with the characteristic 'yoyo' aminotransferase pattern, varying from normal to high over a short timespan. Many of these (approximately 20%) will develop cirrhosis, and a minority will also go on to develop liver cancer.

Differential diagnosis

- As this disease is mainly identified in the chronic phase, other chronic liver diseases should be excluded.

Diagnosis

- Diagnosis is still often clinical because the antibody test gives a high rate of false-positive and false-negative results.
- An antibody (anti-hepatitis C virus) test is available, but only becomes positive several months after the acute infection.

Treatment

- There is accumulating evidence that prolonged courses of alpha-interferon will eradicate chronic infection in a significant proportion of individuals.

Prevention

- The presence of hepatitis C virus is still a major problem for blood transfusion services. Until recently, the UK transfusion services accepted that there was no reliable screening test, whereas in the US large amounts of blood were wasted when aminotransferase levels and anti-HBc were used as surrogate markers of infection. The

anti-hepatitis C virus test is still unhelpful because of the low
sensitivity and specificity of the test. Nonetheless, it is being used
increasingly to try and identify infected blood.

Hepatitis D (delta virus)

Causative agent

● Hepatitis D virus, an incomplete RNA virus.

Epidemiology

● This agent cannot exist without concurrent hepatitis B virus infection
because it needs hepatitis B surface protein to complete its structure.
● Hepatitis D virus is transmitted mainly by the parenteral route, and
in the UK it is seen most commonly in iv drug abusers and haemophiliacs. It is uncommon.
● The epidemiology of the infection elsewhere is not well understood,
although there is some evidence for sexual and mother-to-child
transmission.

Incubation period

● 40–160 days.

Clinical features

● Two clinical patterns are seen. If the delta virus is acquired at the
same time as that for hepatitis B, a severe acute hepatitis ensues with
a high rate of fulminant hepatic failure. Symptoms and signs are as
for hepatitis A virus infection.
● If delta virus infection occurs in a patient who is a chronic hepatitis
B virus carrier, chronic hepatitis D virus infection also follows. There
is often an episode of acute icteric hepatitis at the time of this second
infection, with very aggressive chronic hepatitis ensuing. The majority of chronic hepatitis D virus infections progress to cirrhosis and
death.

Differential diagnosis

● *See* hepatitis A (page 71).

Diagnosis

- Hepatitis D virus infection should be considered in groups at risk, particularly as a cause of severe hepatitis B virus infection or the relapse of chronic hepatitis B.
- The infection can be confirmed by an anti-hepatitis D virus antibody test.

Treatment

- *See* hepatitis B (page 74).

Prevention

- *See* hepatitis B (page 74).

Hepatitis E (epidemic non-A non-B hepatitis)

Causative agent

- Hepatitis E virus, as yet an uncharacterized agent.

Epidemiology

- This infection is seen as a faeco-orally spread disease in many parts of the world, including the Indian subcontinent, Soviet Asia, North Africa and Mexico, but not in the UK.

Incubation period

- 14–63 days.

Clinical features

- The clinical disease is similar to that due to hepatitis A virus infection in all respects, except fulminant hepatitis is more commonly seen, especially in pregnancy.

Differential diagnosis

- As for hepatitis A (page 71).

Diagnosis

- Diagnosis is made by the absence of serological markers for other causes in patients returning from relevant countries with acute hepatitis.

Treatment

- *See* hepatitis A (page 72).

Prevention

- This disease is not prevented by human normal immunoglobulin and travellers should maintain a high level of food and drink hygiene to avoid this and other food and waterborne diseases.

Leptospirosis

Causative agents

- Strains within the *Leptospira interrogans* complex, namely *hebdomadis, canicola, icterohaemorrhagiae* and others. The organism is a spirochaete.

Epidemiology

- The pathogen is found in a variety of wild and domestic animals. The infection may spread to man through contamination of the environment with the animals' urine. *Leptospira* may be ingested or contaminate wounds.
- *Leptospira interrogans* serovar *icterohaemorrhagiae* (the cause of Weil's disease) is an infection of rats, whose urine may contaminate rivers, lakes, sewage pipes and treatment plants putting water sports enthusiasts and sewage workers at particular risk.
- Serovar *canicola* infects dogs and, therefore, potentially their owners.
- Serovar *hebdomadis* is found in cattle and seen as an infection in farm workers and abattoir workers.
- There are 100 cases reported each year in the UK, mostly during the warmer months.

Incubation period

- 7–12 days (range: 2–20).

Clinical features

- Asymptomatic infection is common.
- The illness is often biphasic, commencing with a non-specific 'flu-like illness and fever lasting for 4–7 days. After a short (1–2 days) period of improvement, the more classic features develop including one or some of the features of hepatitis (Weil's disease), meningitis, uveitis/conjunctivitis, rash, and renal impairment, depending on the infecting serovar. Headache is usually intense.
- Examination in the second phase may reveal, in addition to the features of meningitis or hepatitis, a febrile patient with generalized lymphadenopathy, conjunctival injection, myalgia, maculopapular rash and, less commonly, splenomegaly.
- The illness may last up to 30 days and overall the mortality is low (<1%).

Differential diagnosis

- The prodromal illness may be indistinguishable from other non-specific febrile illnesses.
- Other forms of aseptic meningitis can be similar in presentation.
- Leptospirosis should be considered in any patient who is suffering from fever and jaundice at the same time. Cholangitis, malaria, typhoid and EBV-related hepatitis are the only other major causes of this combination.

Diagnosis

- The diagnosis begins with a high index of suspicion if a history of water immersion, sewage contact or at-risk occupation is obtained.
- The organism can be seen in and cultured from blood or CSF specimens during the early phase of the infection, or in a specimen of urine, alkalinized by prior ingestion of potassium citrate, during later stages of the disease, although the yields are poor.
- Serology using an enzyme linked immunoadsorbent assay (ELISA) test for the antibody will retrospectively confirm the diagnosis, although a new IgM test is available.
- Liver and renal function may be abnormal.
- The CSF shows a lymphocytosis, raised protein and normal glucose in meningitis presentations.

Treatment

- Antibiotic therapy with benzylpenicillin 10–20 mg/kg iv or oral tetracyclines 7 mg/kg, 6 hourly, can be effective if given within 4 days of the onset of the prodromal illness. The second phase illness is probably immune mediated and antibiotics are less likely to alter its course.

● Therapy is otherwise supportive.

Prevention

● Groups at risk, including water sports enthusiasts, and farm, sewage and abattoir workers, should be warned of the dangers of this illness. Sewage workers are provided with waterproof clothing and instructed in strict hygiene.

● Doxycycline has been shown to be effective in preventing illness in soldiers training in jungle conditions.

Biliary tract infection (acute cholecystitis and acute cholangitis)

Causative agents

● Enterobacteriaceae.
● Faecal streptococci.
● Anaerobic bacteria.

Epidemiology

● Infection is seen mainly in adults with pre-existing gallbladder and biliary tract disease, including gallstones.

Incubation period

● Unknown.

Clinical features

● Acute cholecystitis presents with right hypochondrial pain, which often radiates to the shoulder or back, fever and, rarely, jaundice. Examination reveals tenderness in the right hypochondrium, fever and a palpable gallbladder in 40%.

● Cholangitis is recognized by the features of Charcot's biliary triad: pain, fever, chills and jaundice. The patient often complains of right hypochondrial pain, which is frequently severe, jaundice, fever up to 40°C and rigors.

● Cholecystitis may progress to empyema of the gallbladder, gallbladder perforation, pancreatitis, cholangitis and septicaemia.

- Cholangitis can be complicated by septicaemia, liver abscess and pancreatitis.

Differential diagnosis

- Cholecystitis must be distinguished from peptic ulcer disease, hepatitis, and non-infectious biliary and gallbladder disease.
- Cholangitis, because of the presence of high fever, should rarely be mistaken for diseases, other than leptospirosis, EBV, hepatitis and in the traveller, malaria and typhoid.

Diagnosis

- This is usually clinical in the case of cholecystitis, although gallstones will be seen on ultrasound. The white blood cell count is usually raised and organisms may be identified on blood culture.
- Cholangitis will be confirmed by a high white cell count on blood film, on 'obstructive' LFTs (high bilirubin and alkaline phosphatase levels), and the responsible organisms found on blood culture. Ultrasound may reveal a gallstone in a dilated common bile duct.

Treatment

- The patient should be hospitalized and given broad-spectrum antibiotics parenterally, including a third generation cephalosporin, an aminoglycoside and metronidazole.
- Some surgeons perform early cholecystectomy in cholecystitis, although many wait until the infection has been treated successfully.
- The biliary tract abnormality leading to cholangitis should be dealt with by, for instance, endoscopic retrograde cholangiography.

Prevention

- These diseases may be prevented by appropriate management of gallstones and biliary tract disease prior to the onset of secondary infection.

CHAPTER 8

Infections of the urogenital system

ALTHOUGH urinary and genital tract infections have very different aetiologies, they are included together because of the similar symptomatology. Urethritis and cystitis can easily be confused, as occasionally can cystitis and pelvic inflammatory disease (PID). The correct diagnosis is particularly important in these common conditions for several reasons.

1 A wide variety of organisms may be responsible in most cases.
2 A definitive diagnosis of sexually transmitted disease (STD) has connotations in terms of the necessary search for associated conditions, such as HIV infection and syphilis, together with contact tracing.

The patient's history, therefore, should not be taken at face value, and a young person with dysuria or vaginal discharge requires very careful examination before a STD is excluded.

Urinary tract infection

Causative agents

● The majority of such infections are caused by *E. coli* although a large range of organisms, including Enterobacteriaceae, *Enterococcus faecalis* and staphylococci, has been implicated. Less commonly, fastidious bacteria have been detected.

Epidemiology

● Between 1 and 3% of children and young adults, and 10 and 20% of the elderly have significant bacteria when randomly tested.
● In childhood, there is a female preponderance (9:1), a significant proportion being related to congenital abnormalities of the urinary tract including urethral strictures and ureteric reflux, although male infections are more common in neonates.
● The female preponderance in young adults is even higher at the age of 10 years (30:1). In the majority, there is no detectable abnormality, but pregnancy and sexual intercourse are significant predisposing features in women.

- The ratio falls to 2:1 female to male as factors including prostatic hypertrophy, neurological disease and general debility contribute to male infection.
- Other significant associations include diabetes, sickle-cell disease and bladder catheterization.

Clinical features

- There are four major syndromes: the urethral syndrome, cystitis, pyelonephritis and asymptomatic bacteriuria.
- The urethral syndrome is a disease of women where a recurrent burning sensation is experienced on passing urine, but pathogenic organisms are not commonly detected and the response to antibiotics is variable. The sufferers sometimes undergo extensive investigation for structural abnormalities which are rarely found. STDs, low-number bacterial infection and lactobacilli are responsible for some cases.
- Cystitis, i.e. infection of the urinary bladder, gives symptoms of suprapubic discomfort, frequency of micturition, dysuria and the production of urine that is cloudy or occasionally bloodstained.
- Pyelonephritis in adults usually includes fever (up to 40°C) and loin pain, which may also be associated with symptoms of cystitis. Urinary tract infection (UTI) in young children and infants is usually of this type, but presents non-specifically with fever, lethargy, vomiting and, less acutely, growth retardation.
- Asymptomatic bacteriuria, defined as the presence of $>10^5$ bacteria/ml of urine of a single organism in the absence of symptoms, is a frequent finding, especially in pregnancy.
- Most of these problems are minor and easily treated with a short course of antibiotics. Cystitis can progress to pyelonephritis. The latter may be complicated by intra-renal and perinephric abscess, septicaemia and renal failure. Stone formation may also be related to urinary infection.
- As UTI in children is commonly associated with ureteric reflux, progressive renal failure is more common.

Differential diagnosis

- Cystitis and urethral syndrome may be difficult to distinguish clinically. Similar symptoms may be produced by urethritis, TB of the urinary tract, malignancy, haematuria and inflammatory conditions involving the urinary tract from without, such as endometriosis.
- Pyelonephritis can sometimes be mistaken for cholecystitis, pneumonia, appendicitis and other abdominal infections.

● The non-specific nature of presentation in infants brings meningitis, pneumonia and a range of causes of growth retardation into the differential diagnosis.

Diagnosis

● Significant infection is confirmed by the finding of $> 10^5$ bacteria/ml of midstream urine in single pure growth. Blood, protein and white cells may also be found, but their presence is not mandatory for the diagnosis. The finding of white cells in the absence of bacteria, if repeatable, may indicate alternative pathology, including TB, urinary tract malignancy or a stone.
● In infants, especially boys, confirmed infection should lead to visualization of the urinary tract. Adults with recurrent infection rarely have detectable abnormalities, although pyelonephritis warrants an ultrasound scan.
● Infection with *Proteus* sp., especially when recurrent, may be associated with a stone in the bladder or kidney.
● In pyelonephritis, the white blood cell count may be raised and organisms cultured from the blood. Renal function tests are only occasionally abnormal.

Treatment

● Lower UTI can usually be eradicated with a single dose of oral antibiotics such as amoxycillin 40 mg/kg or co-trimoxazole 24 mg/kg. It is wise to take a mid-stream urine specimen (MSU) in case of antibiotic resistance in the organism. In difficult cases, antibiotic therapy, guided by cultural findings, may need to be given for a week.
● Pyelonephritis and UTI in young children often requires parenteral antibiotic therapy with a third-generation cephalosporin or aminoglycoside for 7–10 days. If an antibiotic-sensitive organism is found, yet a clinical response is not obtained, a renal abscess should be suspected.
● Non-specific measures, such as increased fluid intake and ingestion or organic acids, may aid recovery.

Prevention

● Children with ureteric reflux and, less commonly, adults with recurrent infection may benefit from long-term prophylactic antibiotics.
● Surgical repair of mechanical abnormalities is at least as important, especially in ureteric reflux where renal damage is probably largely the result of increased pressure within the collecting system.

Acute urethritis

Causative agents

- *Neisseria gonorrhoeae,*
- *Chlamydia trachomatis,*
- *Ureaplasma urealyticum.*
- *Trichomonas vaginalis* and other less common organisms.

Epidemiology

- This syndrome is more common in men than in women.
- In the majority of cases, the organism is sexually transmitted and therefore these infections are seen mainly in young adults.
- The true incidence is unknown, although estimates indicate at least 80 000 cases per year in the UK.
- Associated proctitis and pharyngitis, due to the same organisms, are common and should be sought particularly in homosexual men.

Incubation period

- 2–14 days, although for gonorrhoea it is usually only 4 days.

Clinical features

- Typical features include dysuria and urethral discharge. In gonorrhoea, the discharge is usually purulent, whereas in other causes (non-gonorrhoea urethritis) [NGU] it is frequently mucoid.
- Dysuria is normally present in gonorrhoea, whereas 25% or more cases of NGU do not experience this symptom.
- If untreated, the infection will eventually resolve over weeks or months, although the infected person may remain infectious.
- Complications include epididymitis, prostatitis, urethral stricture, Reiter's syndrome and gonococcal septicaemia (fever, rash, arthralgia/arthritis).

Differential diagnosis

- The symptoms can be mistaken for UTI, especially in women.
- Urethritis may complicate Stevens–Johnson syndrome and post-dysenteric Reiter's syndrome.

Diagnosis

- Diagnosis is achieved by taking appropriate specimens.

1 A direct urethral smear on a microscope slide for Gram-staining and direct observation of a wet preparation (if *Trichomonas* is suspected).
2 A urethral swab in charcoal transport medium for gonococcal culture.
3 Urethral swabs of material for detection of antigens to *Chlamydia* and culture of *Chlamydia*.

- If two specimens of urine are produced at the same time, more mucous strands and white cells in the initial specimen suggest urethritis rather than cystitis.
- Swabs may be taken from the anus, pharynx, and cervix in women.

Treatment

- These conditions are best dealt with at a STD clinic where the tracing of contacts can be performed.
- Gonococcal urethritis responds to procaine penicillin 40 mg/kg with probenecid 15 mg/kg as a single dose in those infected with penicillin-sensitive strains. As resistance is increasing, alternative therapies such as spectinomycin 30 mg/kg given im, a third-generation cephalosporin, or ciprofloxacin may be substituted.
- As co-infection with *Chlamydia* is common, appropriate therapy for that infection should also be given.
- NGU and confirmed infection with *Chlamydia trachomatis* will normally respond to oral tetracycline 7 mg/kg, 6 hourly, for 7 days. Alternatives include oral erythromycin 7 mg/kg, 6 hourly, for 7 days.
- Other organisms require specific therapy, such as metronidazole for *Trichomonas vaginalis*.

Prevention

- Sexual contacts should ideally be treated.
- The use of condoms during intercourse may reduce the risk of spread if the partner is infected.

Genital ulceration, warts and pediculosis

Causative agents

Ulcers

- Herpes simplex type II.
- *Treponema pallidum*.

- *Chlamydia trachomatis.*
- *Haemophilus ducreyi.*
- *Calymmatobacterium granulomatis.*

Warts
- Papilloma virus.
- *Treponema pallidum.*

Pediculosis (crabs)
- *Phthirus pubis.*

Epidemiology

- These conditions are sexually transmitted and therefore are most common in young adults.
- They are particularly common in the tropics, and chancroid (*Haemophilus ducreyi*), lymphogranuloma venereum (LGV) (*Chlamydia trachomatis*) and granuloma inguinale (*Calymmatobacterium granulomatis*) are almost entirely seen as diseases of the traveller from the tropics.

Incubation period

- Herpes simplex: 2–12 days.
- *Treponema pallidum:* 3–90 days
- *Chlamydia trachomatis:* 3–21 days.
- *Haemophilus ducreyi:* 1–14 days.
- *Calymmatobacterium granulomatis:* 8–80 days.
- Papilloma virus: 6–104 weeks.
- *Phthirus pubis:* 7–10 days.

Clinical features

- Genital ulcers vary in size, number and symptoms according to the cause. Features of individual causes are shown in Table 8.1.
- All the lesions will eventually heal spontaneously, but, in chancroid, LGV and granuloma inguinale, extensive local damage may remain.
- Genital warts are usually noticed as painless swellings. Condylomata acuminata (papilloma virus) are pink or grey, sessile or pedunculated and hyperkeratotic. They can be multiple and range in size from 1 to 20 mm. They may be found anywhere over the external genitalia or perineum. The urethra and cervix may also be involved.
- Condyloma lata (secondary syphilis) accompany many of the other manifestations of syphilis at this stage, including generalized rash,

Table 8.1

Disease	Number of ulcers	Morphology of ulcer	Symptoms
Herpes simplex	Often multiple	Small and shallow on genitalia with erythematous surround	Very painful, tender. In primary infection there is fever and tender adenopathy. Recurrent
Primary syphilis (*Treponema pallidum*)	1–2	Clean, indurated on genitalia 5–20 mm	Usually painless and slightly tender
Chancroid (*Haemophilus ducreyi*)	1–10	Ulcerating papules, 1–20 mm, on genitalia. Inguinal adenopathy (50%)	Tender. Secondary infection common
Lymphogranuloma venereum (*Chlamydia trachomatis*)	1	Ulcer is small and transient on genitalia or anus/rectum. Progresses to inguinal adenopathy and suppuration ('bubo')	Fever in majority. Ulcer painless. Rectal disease common
Granuloma inguinale (*Calymmatobacterium granulomatis*)	multiple	Ulcerative nodules on the genitalia (90%) or perineum	Painless, granulomatous, easily bleed

fever and lymphadenopathy. The lesions are found in moist skinfolds including the vulva, scrotum and inner thigh, but also the axillae, breasts and interdigital webs. They are large, painless, moist and grey or red.

- Condylomata acuminata may be symptomless and heal spontaneously, but are associated with anal and cervical carcinoma. Condyloma lata are highly infectious, but heal, along with other manifestations of secondary syphilis, to be succeeded in 30% of cases, by tertiary syphilis months or years later.
- Crab lice may infect axillary, truncal and eyelash hair as well as the pubic area. There is intense itching in these regions, where the organism itself, eggs attached to hair shafts, and small erythematous papules with excoriations may be found.

Differential diagnosis

- Other causes of genital ulceration include trauma, Reiter's syndrome, Behçet's syndrome and HIV seroconversion illness.
- Genital warts may also be caused by molluscum contagiosum, penile pearly papules and skin tumours.
- Scabies and deodorant allergy may be confused with crabs.

Diagnosis

● Investigation of genital ulcers should include the following.

1 Direct microscopy of ulcer exudate by dark-ground microscopy for spirochaetes, Gram-staining for *Haemophilus ducreyi* and Giemsa stain for *Calymmatobacterium granulomatis* and herpes simplex inclusions.
2 Swabs in viral transport medium for herpes simplex, immediate inoculation onto specific media for *Haemophilus ducreyi* and transport in chlamydia media for culture and antigen detection.
3 Non-specific (venereal disease reference laboratory [VDRL] or rapid plasma reagin [RPR]) and specific (treponema pallidum haemagglutination assay [TPHA] or fluorescent treponemal antibody assay [FTA-ABS]) tests will both be positive in late primary syphilis. The specific assays become positive first, although present infection can be serologically confirmed only by positive non-specific tests.

● Condylomata acuminata ulcers are diagnosed by their characteristic appearance. Condylomata lata will be confirmed by the observation of spirochaetes by dark-ground microscopy of exudate and by positive specific and non-specific syphilis serology.
● Crabs and their eggs (nits) are readily recognized by their microscopic appearance.

Treatment

● Herpes simplex: acute attacks respond to topical or oral acyclovir 3 mg/kg 5 times daily for 5 days.
● *Treponema pallidum:* procaine penicillin 20 mg/kg given im daily with probenecid 15 mg/kg orally daily. Alternatives include doxycycline, amoxycillin or a third-generation cephalosporin.
● *Haemophilus ducreyi:* erythromycin 7 mg/kg, 6 hourly, for 7 days is effective, as is co-trimoxazole or cefotaxime
● *Calymmatobacterium granulomatis:* chloramphenicol 7 mg/kg, 6 hourly, or gentamicin 1 mg/kg, 12 hourly, for 3 weeks are most effective, although tetracycline, erythromycin and co-trimoxazole can also be used.
● *Phthirus pubis:* this responds to the application of topical insecticides, including malathion, pyrethrum, permethrin and lindane, to all areas, except the eyelid, which should be mechanically cleaned followed by petroleum jelly application. Bedding and clothes should be washed.
● Condylomata acuminata may be destroyed by topical podophyllin, cryotherapy, diathermy, surgical removal and intralesional interferon.

Prevention

- Monogamy or sexual abstinence are the only reliable methods of avoiding infection, although the use of condoms may give some protection.
- Recurrent herpes simplex ulcers may be prevented, if troublesome, by prophylactic acyclovir 7 mg/kg given 3 or 4 times a day orally.
- All sexual contacts should be sought and treated.

Vulvovaginitis and pelvic inflammatory disease

Causative agent

Vulvovaginitis

- *Candida* spp. (mainly *albicans*).
- *Trichomonas vaginalis.*
- *Gardnerella vaginalis.*

Pelvic inflammatory disease

- *Neisseria gonorrhoeae.*
- *Chlamydia trachomatis,*
- Enterobacteriaceae.
- Faecal streptococci.
- Anaerobic bacteria.

Epidemiology and pathophysiology

- Candida infections (thrush) are common in postpubertal women and complicate antibiotic therapy, diabetes mellitus, pregnancy and oral contraceptive pill use.
- *Gardnerella vaginalis, Trichomonas vaginalis, Neisseria gonorrhoeae* and *Chlamydia trachomatis* are sexually transmitted and seen mainly in young adult women. They are frequently carried asymptomatically.
- Enterobacteriaceae, faecal streptococci and anaerobic infections most commonly follow pregnancy, gynaecological surgery or the use of an intra-uterine contraceptive device.
- Candida infection usually develops during antibiotic therapy.

Incubation period

- *Trichomonas vaginalis:* 5–28 days.
- *Gardnerella vaginalis:* unknown
- *Neisseria gonorrhoeae* and *Chlamydia trachomatis:* 2–14 days.

Clinical features

- In both syndromes, vaginal discharge and dyspareunia are common features.
- In vulvovaginitis, the first symptom noted is pruritus or burning of the vulva and vagina. In candida and trichomonas infections, this is often intense and associated wih dysuria and low (vaginal) dyspareunia; that associated with *Gardnerella vaginalis* is usually mild.
- The associated discharge can be distinctive. In candida infection, it is often sparse, thick and has a consistency like 'curd cheese'. When *Trichomas vaginalis* is the responsible pathogen, the discharge can be copious, yellow and frothy. However, 25% of infections will not produce a vaginal discharge. The fluid discharged on infection with *Gardnerella vaginalis* is frequently sparse, thin and sometimes frothy. There may be a distinctive fishy smell, especially on mixing the fluid with 10% KOH solution. These descriptions should be used as guidelines; there are no hard and fast rules.
- Examination may reveal vulvovaginal redness, although this is uncommon with *Gardnerella vaginalis* infection.
- The presentation of PID, defined here as infection of the uterus or Fallopian tubes, can be variable. If vaginal discharge is present, it suggests an associated cervicitis, when *Neisseria gonorrhoeae or Chlamydia trachomatis* should be particularly suspected. Fever is variable, but frequently high, especially in accute infection. There may be lower abdominal or pelvic pain, which can vary with the menstrual cycle, and dyspareunia is described as being deep inside the pelvis.
- On examination, there is frequently suprapubic tenderness, and discomfort on both cervical ballottement and palpation of the vaginal fornices. The cervix, seen through a vaginal speculum is often reddened from the os outwards, and an endocervical discharge may be observed, particularly in relation to *Chlamydia trachomatis* and *Neisseria gonorrhoeae* aetiologies.
- PID may progress to pelvic abscess formation in the short term and in the long term damage of the Fallopian tubes with infertility, dyspareunia and dysmenorrhoea.
- Gonococcal septicaemia, with fever, rash and arthritis, is occasionally seen.

Differential diagnosis

- Less common causes of vaginitis include foreign bodies within the vagina (especially in children), threadworms, malignant growths, atrophic vaginitis of the elderly and infrequently infections of other types.

- The discharge of endocervicitis can be confused with vaginitis.
- PID can be difficult to distinguish from endometriosis, pelvic appendicitis and inflammation of other pelvic organs, including the rectum and bladder.
- Vaginal discharge in prepubertal girls is sometimes a result of childhood sexual abuse. Otherwise a foreign body should be suspected.

Diagnosis

- In both conditions, a full pelvic examination, including speculum, is mandatory.
- Any vaginal discharge should be examined by microscopy immediately for motile trichomonads, yeasts and 'clue' cells (*Gardnerella vaginalis*) and cultured using appropriate transport media taken for yeasts, trichomonads and *Gardnerella vaginalis*.
- Endocervial swabs should be smeared on a microscope slide for Gram-staining (gonorrhoea) and appropriate specimens sent for gonococcal and *Chlamydia* culture. When STDs are suspected, urethral, rectal and pharyngeal swabs may also be taken.
- Needle aspiration of pelvic contents *per vaginum* may identify faecal and anaerobic organisms as a cause of salpingits, but it is an invasive and painful procedure.
- Gonococcal septicaemia, recognized by the sparse peripheral rash and arthritis, may be confirmed by blood and joint aspiration cultures.

Treatment

- *Candida:* Vaginal pessaries or creams containing clotrimazole or other antifungal preparations. Oral fluconazole 150 mg, or itraconazole 200 mg, 12 hourly, for 2 days are alternatives.
- *Trichomonas vaginalis* and *Gardnerella vaginalis:* both respond to oral metronidazole 3 mg/kg, 8 hourly, for 7 days. Tinidazole is equally effective.
- PID is normally treated with combination therapy, often including a third-generation cephalosporin (e.g. cefotaxime), tetracycline and metronidazole for 10–14 days. Augmentin with metronidazole is a useful alternative. Any intra-uterine contraceptive device is normally removed.
- When *Neisseria gonorrhoeae* is suspected, spectinomycin 30 mg/kg im × 1 with oral doxycycline 1.5 mg/kg, 12 hourly, for 7 days (to cover co-infection with *Chlamydia*) is usually adequate.

Prevention

- *Candida* may be recurrent in the absence of obvious predisposition, in which case an oral agent should be given whilst the sexual partner is also similarly treated. Vaginal instillation of yoghurt may recolonize the vagina with lactobacilli and prevent relapse. Susceptible women may require prophylactic anticandidal therapy if broad-spectrum antibiotics are given.
- STD *may* be prevented by the use of condoms.

CHAPTER 9

Infectious diseases of the skin

THE diagnosis of skin infections is not usually a problem. The difficulty arises when considering what type and route of antimicrobial therapy to use. In the more serious infections, such as erysipelas and cellulitis, undertreatment has often led to increased morbidity. High-dose or iv therapy should always be considered. In the case of uncomplicated wound contaminations, oral or topical antibiotics have little place; antiseptics are the main therapeutic agent.

However, parasitic infections can be easily misdiagnosed, especially scabies, where the typical lesions may not be found. Body lice can also cause a diagnostic problem as these arthropods may not be found readily. As in many infectious diseases, the diagnosis frequently stems from a high level of suspicion of a particular infection. Threadworms, being mainly manifested by skin symptoms, are described in this chapter rather than under gut infections.

Erysipelas, cellulitis and impetigo

Causative agents

Erysipelas
- *S. pyogenes* (Lancefield Group A β-haemolytic streptococci).
- Rarely *Staph. aureus.*

Cellulitis
- *S. pyogenes.*
- *Staph. aureus.*
- Occasionally other organisms.

Impetigo
- *Staph. aureus.*
- *S. pyogenes.*

Epidemiology and pathophysiology

- These infections will be found at any age.
- Erysipelas and cellulitis may follow infection of any skin breach, including chickenpox, leg ulcers, surgical wounds and burns. They

are more common in diabetics, the immunocompromised and the elderly.

- Epidemics due to *S. pyogenes* may be seen in institutions, such as army barracks and old peoples homes.
- Impetigo is a disease mainly found in children, although similar impetiginous lesions occur in adults with secondary infection of skin conditions, such as eczema, psoriasis and insect bites.
- Epidemics of impetigo frequently spread in schools and nurseries.

Incubation period

- 1–3 days.

Clinical features

- **Erysipelas** is an erythematous eruption seen only on the legs and face. After entering the skin through a break that is not always obvious, the streptococcus invades superficial skin layers causing a well-defined, slightly raised, spreading, erythematous plaque with a well-defined edge. It may cover the entire face. There is associated fever and regional lymph node enlargement.
- There may be severe constitutional symptoms. Even after early and adequate therapy, the skin may ulcerate, and healing normally is associated with desquamation.
- Complications may include septicaemia, scarlet fever and glomerulonephritis.
- **Cellulitis** may be confused with erysipelas on a superficial level. The disease represents skin infected through a breach, which in this case is usually obvious, on any part of the body. Tissue invasion is along layers deeper than those involved in erysipelas and results in an erythematous area with ill-defined edges. Fever and regional lymphadenopathy are the rule. Any part of the body can be involved. Ulceration and necrosis may ensue.
- The complications of cellulitis are similar to those of erysipelas except that streptococcal septicaemia is particularly common in cases following infection of surgical wounds. Septicaemia has a 30% mortality.
- **Impetigo** is a disease observed mostly in children and involves exposed areas of skin, especially the face. Starting as small vesicles, the lesions break down to exude pus that dries to form a yellow or gold crust. There may be regional lymphadenopathy but fever and consitutional symptoms are absent. Complications are rare but may include cellulitis and septicaemia. In infants, there can be marked bullous reaction.
- Secondary infection of eczema and other skin lesions with *Staph. aureus* may also produce an impetiginous crust.

Differential diagnosis

- Erysipelas and cellulitis are frequently confused.
- Other similar conditions include Fournier's gangrene – a progressive necrotizing infection of the perineum, gas gangrene – a clostridial infection with gas formation and necrosis, erythrasma – a mild corynebacterial erythematous infection of the groin, and intertrigo, a mixture of infection and oedema of the skinfolds.

Diagnosis

- As erysipelas and cellulitis require urgent therapy with antibiotics (usually given parenterally), an early clinical diagnosis is essential.
- The aetiological agents can be identified by bacterial culture of swabs taken from the rash, nose and throat.
- A high blood white count and rising antistreptococcal antibodies (e.g. ASO titre) may be helpful.

Treatment

- Erysipelas is best treated with high dose benzylpenicillin 40 mg/kg, 6 hourly, iv. Erythromycin may be given to those allergic to penicillin.
- Cellulitis also requires benzylpenicillin (as above), with flucloxacillin 7–14 mg/kg, 6 hourly. If Gram-negative organisms are suspected, such as seen in the immunocompromised or severe burns patients, additional broad-spectrum antibiotic cover, which may have to include therapy for *Pseudomonas aeruginosa*, should be considered.
- Impetigo is best treated with oral flucloxacillin 7 mg/kg, 6 hourly, for 7–10 days or oral erythromycin in the penicillin allergic. Minor lesions may respond to mupirocin or fusidic acid applied topically.

Prevention

- These organisms are infectious and those infected require isolation.
- In institutional outbreaks, which may occur imperceptibly over several months, all patients and staff may require screening for carriage of the organism. Swabs of nose, throat, axillae and perineum are necessary.
- Carriers should be isolated until the organism is eliminated by the use of antiseptics or antibiotics as appropriate.

Furuncles, carbuncles and wound infections

Causative agents

Furuncles (boils) and carbuncles
- Staph. aureus.

Wound infection
- A wide range of Gram-positive and Gram-negative organisms.

Epidemiology and pathophysiology

- Furuncles and carbuncles can occur spontaneously at any age.
- Predisposing factors include diabetes mellitus, immunosuppression and obesity.
- Wounds of any type can become infected, but numerically most important are the chronic leg ulcers seen in the elderly, diabetics and those with venous or arterial insufficiency.
- Wound contamination with MRSA is a particular problem in hospitals where transfer to other patients may lead to a more invasive infection that is difficult to treat.

Clinical features

- A furuncle is an infected hair follicle that presents as a painful nodular lesion. It eventually comes to a head as the overlying skin thins leading to the spontaneous discharge of pus. They are most frequent in moist, hairy areas.
- A carbuncle is a coalition of several infected follicles and is therefore much larger, up to 3 cm, and most commonly found on the nape of the neck where a rubbing collar has allowed entry of the organism. This lesion may cause fever.
- Although resolution is the rule, cellulitis and staphylococcal septicaemia can result from these infections.
- Wounds, including chronic ulcers, are frequently contaminated with organisms. In the majority of cases, such organisms should be seen as harmless commensals, although they may inhibit healing. Infection is indicated by yellow, often malodorous, exudate from the lesion. Organisms of particular concern include *Staph. aureus* (including MRSA) and *S. pyogenes* that may progress to cellulitis and septicaemia. The ulcer may also act as a source of infection to other patients in hospitals and institutions when the two organisms and MRSA, in particular, are a serious threat.

- Infection may, on occasion, contribute to extension of the ulcer when blood supply or immune status is precarious.
- Small furuncles are similar to larger acne lesions or folliculitis (plugging and minor infection of hair follicles).

Diagnosis

- Furuncles and carbuncles are usually so obvious that clinical diagnosis suffices.
- Regular bacteriological swabbing of wounds allows early prescriptive therapy of the complications.

Treatment

- Furuncles can normally be allowed to come to a head and then allowed to burst or are incised. Heat application may hasten this process.
- It is best if carbuncles are surgically incised.
- If there is any evidence of tissue invasion beyond the localized lesion, such as fever or cellulitis, antibiotic therapy in the form of flucloxacillin 7–14 mg/kg, 6 hourly, for 7 days may be prescribed.
- Infected wounds are best treated using the principles of cleaning and drying. This involves cleansing with topical antiseptics until the wound is uninfected, then maintenance cleansing with sterile saline should continue until healing occurs. The wound may be kept dry by air exposure, a loose gauze dressing, or application of absorbent foam or polymer dressings.
- Oral or topical antibiotics have little role in the management of un-complicated wound infections, expect if cellulitis develops.
- Indolent wound infections that seem to be inhibiting healing have been treated, by various exponents, with granulated sugar, honey or golden syrup, or fresh papaya flesh.
- Patients with MRSA in their wounds should, if treated in hospital, be isolated. This is not the case for patients in the community. The carriage of this organism should be managed on the same lines as those for other contaminating organisms. Antibiotics are required only for invasive disease, although urinary carriage *alone* has occasionally been eradicated by rifampicin in combination with other effective antibiotics.
- Recurrent furuncles and carbuncles may necessitate elimination of staphylococcal carriage. This is achieved by identifying the site of carriage by swabbing, and applying topical antiseptics. The skin should also be cleansed with soap followed by antiseptic applications. Clothes must be scrupulously washed.

- In resistant cases, 14 days of flucloxacillin 7 mg/kg, 6 hourly, and rifampicin 10 mg/kg daily, both orally, may eliminate staphylococcal carriage.
- Wounds should be looked after carefully, as described, to prevent new infections.
- Wound infection with MRSA and *S. pyogenes* warrants isolation of patients in hospitals and institutions to prevent spread to others in whom a more invasive illness may develop.

Zoster (shingles)

Causative agent

- Varicella zoster, a herpes virus.

Epidemiology and pathophysiology

- Following an attack of chickenpox, the varicella zoster virus may remain in the sensory nerves and root ganglia and, at a later stage, become reactivated causing the typical rash of zoster which always follows the path of a sensory nerve.
- Although zoster is less infectious, chickenpox can be contracted by susceptible individuals who are in contact. In very rare cases, zoster may be associated with exposure to chickenpox.
- Zoster is more common in the immunocompromised, especially in leukaemia, HIV infection and Hodgkin's disease, which should be considered as an underlying diagnosis, especially in younger people.
- Infants may develop shingles after maternal intra-uterine infection.
- There were 103 deaths attributed to zoster infection in England and Wales and 792 cases per 100 000 population in 1987.

Incubation period

- 1–80 years.

Clinical features

- Burning pain and paraesthesia along the course of a sensory nerve may precede the papular then vesicular rash.
- The rash is distributed along a dermatome.
- The rash is unilateral and never crosses the midline of the body. Disseminated chickenpox lesions may be found, however.

- The vesicles may break down and weep before crusting over, and when the crusts separate from the skin they may leave a depigmented area.
- Ophthalmic zoster, infection of the first division of the trigeminal nerve, may affect the conjunctiva, cornea, sclera or uveal tract, and usually requires specialist ophthalmic assessment.
- Zoster of the maxillary division of the trigeminal nerve causes a unilateral eruption on the cheek and on the same half of the palate.
- Ramsay – Hunt syndrome may be due to involvement of the geniculate ganglion and presents with vesicles in the external auditory meatus and lower motor neurone unilateral facial paralysis (VII nerve palsy).
- The commonest complications are secondary infection with *Staph. aureus* and *S. pyogenes*. Post-herpetic neuralgia affects 50% or more of the elderly with shingles and produces severe stabbing pains over the dermatome which may last up to a year.
- Other complications include meningitis and encephalitis, myelitis, lower neurone paralysis and disseminated zoster in the immuno-compromised. Second and third attacks are occasionally observed.

Differential diagnosis

- Other vesicular rashes, such as eczema herpeticum, when discrete and unilateral, may mimic shingles.

Diagnosis

- The diagnosis is usually clinical.
- The virus can be cultured from vesicular fluid in case of doubt.

Treatment

- In immunocompromised patients, acyclovir 10 mg/kg, 8 hourly, iv for 7–10 days is required. Additional zoster immunoglobulin may help in resistant cases.
- Topical idoxuridine, when continuously applied (e.g. on gauze swabs), or oral acyclovir, 11 mg/kg 5 times daily for 5 days, may shorten the duration of the illness and possibly diminish the incidence of post-herpetic neuralgia if given before the rash is fully erupted in the immunocompetent patient.
- Oral analgesics are often required. Post-herpetic neuralgia may also require amitriptyline up to 75 mg daily or carbamazepine up to 400 mg, 6 hourly.

● Antibacterial agents may be required (e.g. flucloxacillin) for secondary infections.

Prevention

● Patients known to have chickenpox or shingles should be isolated from immunocompromised patients, and pregnant women especially.
● Zoster immunoglobulin may be administered to these groups at risk (see above) within 72 hours of contact with zoster.
● The dose is as follows.

0– 5 years:	250 mg.
6–10 years:	500 mg.
11–14 years:	750 mg.
Older than 15 years:	1 g.

● Neonates whose mothers develop varicella within 6 days of birth of after delivery should also be given immunoglobulin.

Ectoparasite infections (scabies, lice, fleas)

Causative agents

● Scabies: *Sarcoptes scabiei*, a mite.
● Lice: *Pediculus humanis* var. *capitis* (head lice) or *Pediculus humanis corporis* (body lice). See also crab lice, Chapter 7.
● Flea: *Pulex irritans* (human flea).

Epidemiology

● Scabies is more common in poor, overcrowded conditions, but no-one is entirely immune. The infection is spread by close intimate contact.
● Head lice are particularly common in children, especially those with long hair. All socio-economic classes are at risk. Epidemics in schools are frequently observed as the lice are transferred by close contact, combs and brushes.
● Body lice are seen only in circumstances of poverty and poor hygiene. The lice live on clothes, transferring to the human body only to feed. They are transmitted by close contact and the lice may themselves transmit diseases, such as epidemic typhus and relapsing fever.
● Fleas live mainly in furniture, carpets and possibly clothes, passing to the host to feed.

Incubation period

- Scabies: 4–6 weeks.
- Lice: 6–15 days.

Clinical features

- Scabies presents as an intensely itchy rash, especially bad at night. The lesions, which can be vesicular or papular, sometimes with a short burrow leading into them, can be found in the finger-web spaces, arms, legs peri-umbilical area, buttocks and penis, in particular. The symptoms can be persistent and increase in intensity over several weeks. Many family members may be infected.
- The lesions are occasionally extensive, hypertrophic and crusted, so-called 'Norwegian scabies'.
- Secondary infection is common.
- Head lice may often be asymptomatic, but mostly present with itching of the scalp. Sometimes an itchy rash, due to hypersensitivity, may be found elsewhere on the body.
- Inspection of the scalp may reveal the adult lice, which are 1–2 mm in length, or the eggs ('nits') attached to hair shafts.
- Body lice produce an itchy rash, mainly on the trunk, which is macular or papular. Excoriations and secondary infection leading to impetiginous exudates may be seen. These may be extensive and associated with thickened skin from chronic scratching ('vagabonds disease').
- Fleas bite the host leaving a central papule and erythematous halo. Bites can be single or multiple.

Differential diagnosis

- Scabies and body lice may be superficially similar but finding typical lesions help to differentiate the two. Other itchy rashes, such as allergic reactions, may cause confusion. In the traveller returned from West Africa and South America, in whom scabies can be common, onchocerciasis must be considered.
- Head lice can be confused with allergies to shampoo and other scalp applications.
- Bites similar to those of human fleas may be caused by cat and dog fleas, mosquitoes and bedbugs.

Diagnosis

- Scabies is confirmed by finding a typical lesion and removing the contents of a papule/vesicle onto a microscope slide where the adult, eggs or excreta may be seen on microscopy.

- Body lice may be identified on the patient's clothes.
- Head lice or their eggs are normally easily identified on the scalp and hair.
- Fleas may be seen on the furniture, otherwise the diagnosis is clinical.

Treatment

- Scabies is treated with total body applications (except face) of benzyl benzoate on 2 successive days, or lindane once each week for 2 successive weeks. The lotion should be left on for at least 6 hours (usually overnight) after which it is washed off and the bedding and clothes are also washed.
- Symptomatic treatment with antihistamines or 1% hydrocortisone are often required, and the itching may last for many weeks after the infection has been successfully treated.
- Head lice require scalp applications of malathion or carbaryl lotions (not shampoo) left on for 12 hours and shampooed out. The hair may be combed with a nit comb to remove eggs.
- The rash of body lice may require antihistamines or flucloxacillin. The arthropod is destroyed if the clothes are washed in a hot cycle and ironed, or dusted with insecticide such as malathion.
- Flea bites heal after a few days and may require symptomatic relief. Furniture, carpets and clothing suspected to be infected should be treated with insecticides, as should any cats and dogs within the house.

Prevention

- Prevention of infection with body lice and fleas depends on healthy hygienic living conditions.
- Scabies may be difficult to avoid, although infected individuals should ideally be isolated.
- Head lice can be prevented by careful regular head inspection within schools and institutions, and varying the type of insecticide used for therapy in order to avoid the development of resistance.

Threadworm infection

Causative agent

- *Enterobius vermicularis*, a nematode.

Epidemiology and pathophysiology

- The adult female worm, present in the colon and rectum, lays eggs at night around the anus which causes intense peri-anal itching.
- The eggs stick to fingers or nails, which have been used to scratch the irritated peri-anal region, or, less frequently, to bedclothes or dust. The eggs are then ingested by the host or other close contacts.
- The eggs mature into larvae in the intestine, and eventually into adult worms which then continue the cycle.
- Up to 20% of children in Britain will at some time be infected. The commonest age being 5–14 years.

Incubation period

- 36–53 days.

Clinical features

- Marked peri-anal itching, particularly at night, is the main symptom. Perineal and vaginal irritation may also be a feature in young children.
- White thread-like worms are often seen in the faeces or peri-anal region.
- Threadworm infestations are sometimes found in appendices removed at operation.

Differential diagnosis

- Any other cause of peri-anal itching, such as eczema, psoriasis or deodorant allergy, must be excluded.

Diagnosis

- The worms may be seen in the faeces.
- Ova may be detected by applying the adhesive surface of sellotape to the peri-anal skin first thing in the morning and examining this under a microscope.

Treatment

- Mebendazole (100 mg × 2), each dose separated by 2-week intervals for *everyone in the family* over 3 years old.
- Piperazine 50–75 mg/kg orally every day for 7 days is suitable for young children.

- The family should be encouraged to wash their hands, cut their nails and use a nailbrush after toilet use and before meals for the 2 weeks of therapy.

Prevention

- Treat the whole family.
- Strict personal hygiene will prevent spread.

Superficial mycoses

Causative agents

- *Trichophyton* spp.
- *Microsporum* spp.
- *Epidermophyton* spp.

Epidemiology and pathophysiology

- Zoophilic infections are acquired from animal sources. Cattle ringworm (*Trichophyton verrucosum*) and dog ringworms (*Microsporum canis*) are the commonest.
- Geophilic fungi, acquired from soil, are uncommonly the cause of disease.
- Anthropophilic fungi, including *Trichophyton rubrum* (tinea pedis and tinea cruris), *Trichophyton interdigitale* (tinea pedis) and *Epidermophyton floccosum* (tinea cruris), are organisms that naturally infect man and spread readily from person to person, e.g. tinea pedis acquired at swimming pools.

Incubation period

- Largely unknown, but probably 1–2 weeks.

Clinical features

- The lesion usually has a raised edged, and is circular and scaly, although there are exceptions depending on pathogen and site of infection.
- Tinea pedis (athlete's foot) starts in the interdigital spaces or plantar surface of the toes; the infection causes scaling, cracking and itching. Spread to the sole of the foot and the formation of bullae may occur in infections with *Trichophyton rubrum* and *Trichophyton interdigitale*, respectively.

- Infection can be prolonged, recurrent or complicated by cellulitis.
- Tinea corporis represents classic ringworm, producing the typical circular, raised edge, flat centred, flaky lesions varying in diameter from a few millimetres to several centimetres. In some cases, the area may be very inflamed and pustular, as is seen in infections related to *Microsporum canis* and *Trichophyton verrucosum*. Most cases are zoophilic and can occur anywhere on the body including the face.
- Tinea cruris is a scaly, itchy lesion starting in the groin and spreading to adjacent areas; it is often bilateral. It is mainly an infection of young men due to anthropophilic agent such as *Trichophyton rubrum*.
- Tinea manuum is mainly an infection of the palm, otherwise it is similar to tinea pedis.
- Tinea barbae, an involvement of the beard and surrounding area, is often due to *Trichophyton verrucosum* and therefore frequently pustular.
- Tinea capitis describes scalp infection with inflammation, scaling and hair loss. In some cases, pus and exudate form an overlying mass, the so-called kerion. The majority of cases occur in children. Most lesions eventually heal.
- Nail infection presents as sub-ungual inflammation with nail distortion and thickening.

Differential diagnosis

- The most common conditions to be confused are eczema (dermatitis) and psoriasis. In more pustular lesions, bacterial infection may be suspected.
- Erythrasma due to the bacterium *Corynebacterium minutissimum* and candida infection of the groin are similar to tinea cruris, although the latter will have recognizable satellite lesions. Both are sensitive to clotrimazole cream.
- Seborrhoeic dermatitis and alopecia areata are to be distinguished from tinea capitis and nail infections may be mimicked by *Candida*, trauma and psoriatic lesions.

Diagnosis

- Definitive diagnosis can be confirmed by examining skin scrapings or nail clippings, after preparation with potassium hydroxide for fungal hyphae. Culture in Sabouraud's medium will aid further identification.
- Some fungi causing tinea capitis will fluoresce under ultraviolet (UV) (Wood's) light.

Treatment

- Keratolytic agents, such as Whitfield's ointment, applied thrice daily to hyperkeratotic lesions that are well-defined, are messy but effective agents.
- Topical creams containing one of the azole antifungal agents applied once or twice daily are convenient and effective for most lesions over 2–6 weeks. Tinea pedis and nail infections can be difficult, requiring prolonged or alternative therapies.
- Systemic agents, such as griseofulvin and ketoconazole, may be used for extensive, rapidly spreading or invasive infections, although they can have severe side-effects.
- Newer drugs such as fluconazole, terbinafine and itraconazole show promise.

Prevention

- Zoophilic infections may be prevented by avoiding close contact with animals.
- Tinea pedis can be avoided by the use of footwear in the swimming-pool surrounds.

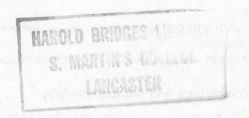

CHAPTER 10

Infections in and around the eye

THERE are few more worrying presentations in medicine than the painful red eye. The diagnosis is most likely to be conjunctivitis, which will resolve quickly, but occasionally a more serious disease underlies the symptoms. If the latter is misdiagnosed, the patient's eyesight rapidly becomes at risk. There can usually be little doubt about the diagnosis of orbital cellulitis, and the major problem arises in getting the patient to hospital fast enough for iv antibiotics and ancillary therapy to prevent progression and permanent damage. If there is any doubt, expert opinion should be sought without delay.

Conjunctivitis

Causative agents

Bacteria
- *S. pneumoniae.*
- *H. influenzae.*
- *Staph. aureus.*
- *Neisseria gonorrhoeae.*
- *Chlamydia trachomatis.*
- *Pseudomonas aeruginosa.*

Viruses
- Adenoviruses and enteroviruses are the major cause of primary infection.
- Herpes simplex should always be considered.

Epidemiology and pathophysiology

- Epidemics of viral conjunctivitis, especially adenovirus, are frequently observed. Most causes of primary viral conjunctivitis are highly infectious.
- Viruses account for 20% of cases.
- Bacterial conjunctivitis is the most common cause and is usually seen sporadically. Pseudomonas infection arises from contaminated contact lenses and eyedrops.
- Conjunctivitis in infants is notifiable and may be acquired from the female genital tract and recurrent infections may indicate teaduct abnormalities.

Incubation period

● Varies, but is usually very short.
● 7–14 days for adenovirus infection.

Clinical features

● In adults, the infection presents with itching or pain, conjunctival
injection and a discharge. The fluid may be clear or purulent, often
crusting on the eyelids. In severe infections, the conjunctiva may
become oedematous and thickened. The conjunctival erythema is
diffuse and involves the conjunctival surfaces of the eyelids.
Occasionally papillae may form.
● Adenovirus infection may cause a typical syndrome of pharyngitis,
fever and lymphadenopathy in addition to the conjunctivitis
(pharyngoconjunctival fever). A more serious form of this disease
with keratitis leading to severe eye pain and photophobia ('epidemic'
keratoconjunctivitis) can occur. These illnesses last 7–14 days.
● Apart from adenovirus syndromes, and the rare cases due to herpes
simplex which progress to corneal ulceration, a clinical aetiological
diagnosis is usually not possible.
● In infants, underlying causes include venereal disease of the mother
(*Chlamydia trachomatis* or *Neisseria gonorrhoeae*) and should be kept in
mind. In recurrent infections, a blocked tearduct is often to be found.
● Complications are uncommon in adult infection, except in herpes
simplex or severe bacterial infection, although untreated bacterial
infections can be prolonged. Viral infections normally resolve within
1 week.
● Infant infection is again usually uncomplicated, although progression
to keratitis and corneal damage is occasionally seen.

Differential diagnosis

● There are numerous, sometimes very serious, causes of the painful
red eye. These include glaucoma, keratitis and anterior uveitis. If in
doubt, urgent ophthalmological opinion should be sought. *In general*,
the more serious illnesses do not produce erythema spreading to the
conjunctiva under the eyelid and the pain and photophobia are
usually more severe.
● Conjunctivitis may be a manifestation of many generalized infections
and non-infectious diseases. These include measles, chickenpox,
toxic shock syndrome, Reiter's disease, Stevens–Johnson syndrome
and allergy, including 'hay fever'.

Diagnosis

- Diagnosis depends on the recognition of clinical features not in keeping with a more severe, deep-seated problem.
- The organisms can be isolated from swabs taken in suitable viral chlamydial and bacterial transport media.
- In severe conjunctivitis, it is wise to stain the cornea with fluorescein and examine under blue light for evidence of herpes simplex infection with associated dendritic ulceration.

Treatment

- Most cases of presumed viral aetiology settle with mild analgesia and the use of dark glasses.
- When bacterial infection is likely, topical chloramphenical eyedrops 0.5% starting 2 hourly with additional ointment at night is usually successful.
- Tetracycline (1%) ointment applied twice daily for 5 days plus erythromycin 7–15 mg/kg orally every 6 hours for 2 weeks is required for chlamydia infection.
- Neonatal gonococcal conjunctivitis requires parenteral penicillin or cephalosporin.
- Infants with recurrent infections require investigation for lacrimal duct obstruction.
- Steroid eyedrops should never be given unless it is certain that herpes simplex infection is not present. This infection responds to topical acyclovir 3% applied 5 times daily and continued for at least 3 days after cure.

Prevention

- Pregnant mothers at risk of sexually acquired diseases may be screened before going into labour.
- When *Chlamydia* or *Neisseria gonorrhoeae* are found in an infant, the parents must be screened and treated.
- Viral conjunctivitis is highly infectious in many cases and reducing contact with the infected person may reduce the risk of transmission.

Keratitis (corneal inflammation)

Causative agents

- Bacteria: *Staph. aureus, S. pneumoniae, Pseudomonas aeruginosa* and others.

- Viruses: herpes simplex, adenoviruses.
- Fungi have also been implicated.
- Acanthamoeba.

Epidemiology and pathophysiology

- The conjunctiva acts as a protective layer over the cornea and therefore must be breached before keratitis occurs.
- Keratitis follows conjunctivitis, trauma and may also be seen in diabetics and the immunosuppressed.

Incubation period

- 1–14 days.

Clinical features

- The pain of keratitis is usually severe and exacerbated by eye and eye-lid movements. Vision may be blurred and discharge slight or absent. Photophobia and blepharospasm are also frequently found.
- Examination often reveals corneal turbidity, dilation of vessels around the edge of the cornea ('ciliary flush'), and in severe cases, corneal ulceration revealed by fluorescein and blue light.
- Complications include corneal perforation and pus formation seen as a fluid level in the anterior chamber in front of the iris ('hypopyon'). Endophthalmitis and loss of vision may ensue rapidly.

Differential diagnosis

- Severe conjunctivitis and other causes of the painful red eye, such as glaucoma, may cause confusion.
- Keratitis may be seen during the course of systemic disease, such as chickenpox, ophthalmic shingles (when the side of the nose is involved), syphilis, Reiter's syndrome and vitamin A deficiency.

Diagnosis

- The diagnosis must be suspected in the groups at risk, particularly after recent eye trauma, however minor.
- Bacteriological swabs and scrapings should be taken from the cornea, as should viral swabs when a virus is the suspected pathogen.
- This condition can quickly deteriorate and usually requires treatment by an ophthalmic surgeon.

Treatment

- In addition to symptomatic relief, therapy usually involves topical and parenteral antibiotics appropriate to the suspected organism.
- Adenoviral keratitis resolves without antimicrobial therapy.
- Topical steroids have a role, as long as herpes simplex infection with corneal ulceration has been ruled out. Pupillary dilations may prevent adhesions to the iris (synechiae).

Prevention

- Potential causes of eye trauma such as entropion, incorrect contact lens use and chronic dry eyes should be dealt with appropriately.

Infections of the tissues surrounding the eye

Causative agents

Eyelid infection
- *Staph. aureus* in the majority.

Teargland infection
- *Staph. aureus.*
- *H. influenzae.*
- *Streptococcus* spp.

Orbital cellulitis
- *Staph. aureus.*
- *S. pyogenes.*
- *S. pneumoniae.*
- *H. influenzae.*

Epidemiology and pathophysiology

- Infections of the eyelid usually arise spontaneously but especially in the case of blepharitis, associated seborrhoeic dermatitis and mascara use have been implicated.
- The tear gland is rarely infected, but trauma and bacteraemia occasionally lead to this problem. Tearduct obstruction and infection is dealt with under 'conjunctivitis' (*see* page 108).
- Orbital cellulitis most commonly follows sinusitis, but also less frequently it is the result of local trauma or bacteraemia.

Incubation period

● 1–14 days.

Clinical features

● Eyelid infections include blepharitis – an inflammation of the lid margins which can be acute or chronic, a sty – an infected sebaceous or meibomian gland, and chalazion – a non-infectious granulomatous inflammation of a meibomian gland, which is occasionally secondarily infected. Sties and chalazions produce eyelid swellings. In the former, there is redness and pain until the small abscess 'points' along the lid margin. A chalazion is a swelling towards the lid centre which is smooth, round and non-tender unless secondarily infected. These conditions will usually resolve; in the case of sties, after discharge of the contents.
● Tear gland infection is rare but presents as a painful swelling of the gland in the upper outer eyelid. An abscess may occasionally track to other nearby structures.
● Orbital cellulitis is a severe and potentially life-threatening infection. The eyelids on one side are swollen and tender, with great difficulty in opening the eye. The patient is feverish and complains of pain around the eye. If the eyelids are separated the eye may be seen to be infected and pushed forward. Additional signs of sinusitis may be present as well as a nasal discharge.
● Orbital cellulitis may progress to abscess formation within the orbit, cavernous sinus thrombosis, osteomyelitis, cerebral abscess and blindness.

Differential diagnosis

● Infective blepharitis needs to be distinguished from blepharitis due to dermatitis.
● Sties and chalazions can occasionally be mimicked by other tumours of the lids.
● Orbital cellulitis may be mistakenly diagnosed as cavernous sinus thrombosis, which is an equally serious condition. Fungal infections of the orbit, or orbital osteomyelitis and severe allergic phenomena with eyelid involvement may also present in a similar fashion.

Diagnosis

● Eyelid and tearduct infections are usually diagnosed clinically. Swabs for culture are occasionally helpful.

- Orbital cellulitis is confirmed by the typical clinical features, a high blood white count and X-ray evidence of sinusitis.
- Bacteriological specimens may be taken from the eye, nose, sinuses (by puncture) and blood.
- CT, when available, may also show typical features of orbital cellulitis.

Treatment

- Blepharitis will respond to topical antibiotics or antibiotic/steroid combinations.
- Sties and infected chalazions do not need antibiotic therapy, but sties can come to a head more quickly with a warm compress. Antibiotic drops or ointment may prevent spread of infection to adjacent glands.
- Teargland infection requires systemic antibiotics.
- Orbital cellulitis requires broad-spectrum antibiotic therapy with, for instance, cefotaxime 50 mg/kg iv every 8 hours with flucloxacillin 15 mg/kg, 6 hourly. Sinus drainage may also be required.

Prevention

- None of these conditions are preventable.

CHAPTER 11

The exanthemata, infection-related rashes and childhood infectious diseases

THESE conditions are grouped together because they are mainly diseases of childhood. Most of them can be prevented by appropriate vaccination and, in many cases, are now seen less frequently. There is therefore a risk that doctors may fail to recognize what used to be common illnesses.

Adults unlucky enough to be non-immune can also be infected, and such diseases are often severe with a high morbidity and, sometimes, mortality. It is important not only to be able to recognize the diseases whilst they still exist, but also to continue to encourage vaccination and thereby reduce their incidence.

Although the specific therapies of these diseases are important, it must be remembered that young children are especially prone to febrile convulsions. Particular attention should be paid to keeping the child cool by the use of paracetamol, cool air and fanning, and tepid sponging.

Chickenpox (varicella)

Causative agent

● Varicella zoster, a herpes virus, which also causes herpes zoster or shingles.

Epidemiology and pathophysiology

● Commonly affects children between the ages of 5 and 9 years.
● 1304 cases per 100 000 population were recorded in England and Wales in 1987.
● Only 5% of adults are without immunity.
● Usually a minor self-limiting illness, but it can be fatal, especially in adults; 24 deaths occurred in England and Wales in 1987.
● Patients are infective from 2 days before the appearance of the rash until all the lesions are crusted, although most spread occurs whilst the rash is appearing.
● It is highly contagious and mainly spread by droplet transmission; less commonly, it may be spread by virus shed from the skin.

● Transplacental transmission occurs and can lead to congenital abnormalities, although this is less frequent than is seen with rubella. Recent evidence suggests there may be no rash even when infection has occurred *in utero*.

Incubation period

● Usually 14–17 days, although it can be up to 21 days.

Clinical features

● A short prodromal period may be seen, usually in adults, with malaise, fever, headache, and cough.
● The rash begins with a crop of papules which quickly become vesicular. Vesicles then become pustules which either disappear or heal with crusting. Lesions often continue to appear for up to 5 days with the fever persisting.
● The rash is usually centripetal, i.e. mainly affecting the trunk with less on the limbs. The scalp will also be involved.
● Vesicles are usually found also on the mucus membranes, especially in the mouth.
● Although principally a childhood disease, it may also affect adults, in whom the symptoms are often more severe.
● The commonest complication is secondary staphylococcal infection of the vesicles.
● Other complications include the following.

1 **Encephalitis**, which is more common in children. Up to 0.2% of children develop fits, focal neurological signs and clouding of consciousness. There is an associated morbidity and mortality of 5–20%. This can be seen up to 4 weeks after the acute infection.
2 **Cerebellar ataxia** can also occur at any time during the first 21 days, but it normally resolves without harm within 2–4 weeks. Optic neuritis, myelitis and meningitis are other rare sequelae.
3 **Pneumonitis** is uncommon in children, but X-ray abnormalities develop in up to 20% of adults. Fever, cough, dyspnoea, haemoptysis and chest pain may all be features of this frequently devastating complication.

● During pregnany, chickenpox may affect the fetus. Associated fetal abnormalities include limb hypoplasia, cerebral atrophy, choroidoretinitis, optic atrophy, fits, skin lesions and psychomotor retardation. Congenital chickenpox is rare, due to the high level of immunity usually found in pregnant mothers. Infection late in pregnancy may cause the child to be born with, or develop soon after birth, a chickenpox rash, which is potentially very serious.

- Chickenpox in the immunocompromised is life-threatening, causing death in about 15%.
- Haemorrhagic chickenpox occurs when bleeding takes place into the vesicles and is related to thrombocytopenia or disseminated intravascular coagulation.
- Other complications include hepatitis, arthritis, nephritis, myocarditis, venous thrombosis and corneal lesions.

Differential diagnosis

- This includes eczema herpeticum, Stevens–Johnson syndrome, and Coxsackie virus infection.

Diagnosis

- A clinical diagnosis usually suffices.
- Virus can be grown from the vesicle.
- Serology reveals a rise in antibody titres.

Treatment

- Symptomatic therapy alone is required, except in severe cases and the immunocompromised when acyclovir, 10 mg/kg iv, 8 hourly, for 5–10 days may be used.
- Antibiotics, particularly flucloxacillin are required for bacterial superinfection.

Prevention

- A live attenuated vaccine is being investigated.
- Zoster-specific immunoglobulin may be essential in immunocompromised patients who have been exposed to the virus. It may also be considered in pregnant mothers known to have been in contact with varicella and who are not immune, and for infants born to mothers who develop chickenpox within 5 days of delivery.

Rubella (German measles)

Causative agent

- A rubivirus.

Epidemiology and pathophysiology

● It is infective from 1 week before until 4 days after the rash.
● It is droplet spread, but the virus is also excreted in the urine and can cross the placenta.
● It most commonly affects children aged 4–9 years especially in the spring.
● The likelihood of congenital rubella syndrome developing during a non-immune pregnancy is at its highest in the first 4 weeks of the pregnancy (50%), falling to 25% in weeks 4–8 and 10% in weeks 8–12.
● The incidence was 624 cases per 100 000 population in England and Wales in 1987; 11 482 were notified in 1990.

Incubation period

● 14–21 days.

Clinical features

● The illness is characterized by a transient discrete, fine, maculopapular, erythematous rash starting on the face, and is often accompanied by postauricular and occipital lymphadenopathy, and fever. These last for up to 5 days but are usually mild.
● Pharyngitis and conjunctivitis are common. However, approximately 50% of infections are asymptomatic.
● Complications include arthritis, thrombocytopenia and encephalitis (1 in 6000 cases).
● Congenital rubella syndrome may occur if the fetus is infected especially during the first 4 months of pregnancy.
● The commonest manifestations of congenital rubella syndrome are deafness, cataract, glaucoma, heart defects and mental retardation in 50% or more. Microcephaly (20%), microphthalmia (18%), jaundice (15%), pneumonia (15%), hepatomegaly (64%), splenomegaly (58%), low birthweight (60%), and radiological bone lesions (30%) may also be found.

Differential diagnosis

● The rash may be confused with measles, scarlet fever, entero- and parvovirus infections, and roseola infantum.

Diagnosis

● Suspected cases of rubella, especially during the first trimester of pregnancy, should be notified to the obstetrician and arrangements made for sera to be taken to look for rubella specific IgM, which is present in recent infection.

Treatment

● Symptomatic treatment alone suffices for most cases.
● Termination of pregnancy may be offered to a woman who is known to have contracted rubella during the pregnancy.

Prevention

● Rubella is part of the MMR vaccination given to infants around 15 months of age or at pre-school booster.
● Monovalent rubella vaccination will continue to be given to teenage girls whilst MMR uptake increases.
● The rubella component of the vaccine is 95% effective in producing an appropriate antibody response.
● Vaccination should be avoided during pregnancy, and seronegative women found during pregnancy should be offered vaccination after delivery but before discharge home.

Measles

Causative agent

● Rubeola virus, a paramyxovirus.

Epidemiology and pathophysiology

● Measles is infectious from a few days before the onset of the rash to 2 days after the rash has appeared.
● It is droplet spread and highly infectious.
● Children are most commonly infected.
● Incidence: 82 061 in 1986; 42 165 in 1987; 85 642 in 1988; 23 565 in 1989; and 13 291 in 1990 – this latest drop in reported cases may be due to the introduction of MMR vaccine.

Incubation period

● 10–14 days.

Clinical features

- The prodromal illness begins with a fever, cough, runny nose and conjunctivitis lasting for 1–3 days.
- Koplik's spots, small, white papules on the buccal mucosa, may be apparent at this stage, but may disappear once the cutaneous rash has appeared.
- Following the prodromal illness the characteristic rash appears. It is maculopapular, red, and becomes confluent, starting at the ears and spreading down to the trunk. Desquamation may be seen in severe cases. Fever, conjunctivitis, cough and runny nose continue during the phase of exanthem.
- Complications are common and include otitis media, croup, bronchitis, bacterial pneumonia and convulsions. Rarely, encephalitis, which has an incidence of 1 in 5000 reported cases, and pneumonitis have been seen.
- Subacute sclerosing panencephalitis, characterized by mental deterioration, fits and, ultimately, death, may be a late complication of measles, occurring 1–18 years after the initial infection. An estimated 10 deaths per year occur due to this complication in the UK, although its incidence has rapidly fallen since the introduction of immunization.

Differential diagnosis

- A mild disease may be confused with rubella or parvovirus infection.
- Drug rashes, in particular the ampicillin reaction in infections with EBV, are similar to measles, as occasionally is the rash of Kawasaki disease.

Diagnosis

- This is almost entirely clinical.
- Serology can be used to confirm infection by rising antibody titre, but it is seldom necessary.

Treatment

- Symptomatic relief is normally all that is required.
- Antibiotics are required for the 2% with pneumonia and must cover *Staph. aureus*, *S. pneumoniae*, *H. influenzae* and *S. pyogenes*.
- Measles pneumonitis will respond to nebulized ribavirine.

Prevention

● Active immunization is effective against measles as is demonstrated in countries where measles immunization is mandatory before school entry, e.g. the USA.
● Measles is a live vaccine and should be offered (usually in the combined MMR vaccine) to all children between the age of 1 and 2 years for whom there is no valid contraindication (*see* Chapter 17 on immunization).
● The vaccine confers protection in about 95% of children for at least 25 years, and perhaps even life long.
● In 1986, the measles vaccination uptake rate was 71% overall, throughout the country, although there was enormous regional variation.
● Post-exposure prophylaxis for measles – single-antigen measles or MMR vaccine can be used for prophylaxis after exposure to measles. It must be given within 72 hours of exposure if it is to be effective, and preferably within 48 hours. Human normal immunoglobulin may also offer some protection.

Parvovirus infection (fifth disease, slapped cheek syndrome, erythema infectiosum)

Causative agent

● Human parvovirus B19.

Epidemiology and pathophysiology

● Person-to-person transmission is by droplet.
● It is a common infection in school children, amongst whom outbreaks are frequently seen.
● In serological studies, adults show a high level of past infection (30–60%).

Incubation period

● 4–14 days.

Clinical features

● This infection typically presents in a relatively healthy child with an erythematous facial rash (slapped cheek appearance).

- An erythematous maculopapular, confluent or reticular rash may also be present on the trunk and extremities along with generalized lymphadenopathy and fever.
- The rash may occasionally recur for weeks or months and is sometimes itchy, but the acute illness is normally short (7–10 days).
- Asymptomatic infection is common (approximately 20%).
- A moderately severe self-limiting arthritis of small or medium-sized joints can occur in adults.
- In immunocompromised patients with haematological disease, infection can cause a severe prolonged aplastic anaemia.
- In patients with haemolytic anaemia, such as sickle-cell disease, this virus causes a transient aplastic crisis.
- In pregnancy, fetal infection can occur leading to severe anaemia, congestive heart failure and intra-uterine death (fetal hydrops). However, most women affected with the virus will not have an affected fetus and the calculated risk is less than 10%. Many women over the age of 20 years will have previously been infected with the virus (approximately 60%) and therefore are at minimal risk from infection. If miscarriage or stillbirth does not occur, the infant will be normal at birth.

Differential diagnosis

- Rubella is the exanthem most likely to cause confusion, although measles, roseola infantum and enterovirus infection may also give rise to a similar illness.

Diagnosis

- Diagnosis is usually made on clinical grounds.
- A serological test for IgM antibody will confirm the diagnosis

Treatment

- There is no specific therapy, but the immunocompromised and patients with haemolytic anaemia may require blood transfusion during the period of aplasia.
- Immune serum has been given to the immunocompromised who have chronic anaemia and it seems to be effective.
- Intra-uterine blood transfusion of hydropic fetuses has been successful.

Prevention

- There is as yet no vaccine.
- Children with suspected infection should be isolated from pregnant women.

Roseola infantum (exanthem subitum, sixth disease)

Causative agent

- Human herpes virus type 6 (HHV-6).

Epidemiology and pathophysiology

- It is seen mainly in children under 3 years old.
- It is probably droplet spread.
- Most cases are seen during the spring and autumn.

Incubation period

- Probably 10–15 days.

Clinical features

- The child is febrile for 3–5 days, often with a temperature as high as 40°C, then as the fever subsides a discrete maculopapular rash appears, first on the trunk and then on the face and limbs. There is associated lymphadenopathy.
- Adults may present with a glandular fever-like illness.
- Thrombocytopenia and encephalitis are rare complications.

Differential diagnosis

- Rubella, parvovirus and enterovirus may manifest with a similar rash, but the appearance of rash as the fever subsides is unusual in the other conditions.

Diagnosis

- The serological test is not widely available.

Treatment

● Symptomatic only.

Prevention

● There is no vaccine.

Hand, foot and mouth disease

Causative agents

● Coxsackie virus types A16, (A10 and A5).
● Other Coxsackie viruses may also be implicated.

Epidemiology and pathophysiology

● Enterovirus infections are most common in the late summer and in autumn.
● It is faeco-orally or droplet spread.
● Children below the age of 10 years are most frequently affected.
● This disease is not related to foot and mouth disease of cattle.
● Family outbreaks are frequently seen.

Incubation period

● 3–7 days.

Clinical features

● The disease presents with a fever (up to 39°C), malaise, sore mouth and difficulty in swallowing. It is mild and short-lived.
● Oral vesicles can become ulcers, although they are few in number and seen mostly on the tongue and buccal mucosa.
● Erythematous papules, vesicles or pustules occur on the lips, palms of the hands, and sides and backs of the fingers, or plantar aspect of the foot, in 75% of infections. They are usually painful.
● These lesions fade over 2–3 days.
● Systemic symptoms, such as cough, abdominal pain and diarrhoea, are an occasional accompaniment.
● Rare complications include viral meningitis and a disseminated eruption associated with eczema.

Differential diagnosis

- This includes mild chickenpox, herpangina and herpes simplex infection.

Diagnosis

- The clinical features are usually obvious.
- Coxsackie serology is less reliable.

Treatment

- There is no treatment other than reassurance.

Scarlet fever

Causative agents

- *S. pyogenes* (Lancefield Group A β-haemolytic streptococci)
- Rarely *Staph. aureus*.

Epidemiology and pathophysiology

- This disease is more common in children.
- It is usually droplet spread, although foodborne and milkborne transmission of *S. pyogenes* has been seen.
- 7194 cases were notified in England and Wales in 1990.
- The number of cases notified continues to decline and is currently about 33% of the total 20 years ago.
- The highest rates of infection are amongst 3–6-year-olds.

Incubation period

- 1–7 days.

Clinical features

- Scarlet fever usually begins on the second day of a streptococcal sore throat. The tonsils and fauces may be red, swollen and covered with a patchy white exudate. The cervical glands may be enlarged and tender, and there is a fever up to 40°C.

- The rash of scarlet fever begins as a bright flush starting on the face, but sparing the lips and leaving the so-called circumoral pallor. It spreads downwards on to the trunk and limbs, accompanied by punctuate erythema of the diffuse rash and fine macules on less severely affected skin.
- Skinfold accentuation (Pastia's sign) is prominent.
- The rash fades from above downwards, disappearing after about a week. Fine desquamation follows and particularly involves the hands and feet.
- The white strawberry tongue of scarlet fever is coated with white fur through which enlarged papillae stick out. This is followed the next day by the red strawberry tongue when the white fur peels from the edges and the lip of the tongue inwards leaving prominent papillae on a glazed red surface.
- The more severe form, so-called toxic scarlet fever, is a serious illness in which confusion, hypotension, renal failure, myocarditis and hepatitis can occur.
- Scarlet fever may follow streptococcal infections other than tonsillitis, including skin infections.
- Other complications of infection with *S. pyogenes*, such as septicaemia, rheumatic fever and glomerulonephritis, may accompany scarlet fever.

Differential diagnosis

- The similar rash may be seen in severe rubella infection, staphylococcal toxic shock syndrome and Kawasaki disease.

Diagnosis

- The organism is readily cultured from swabs of the throat or other infected sites.
- An ASO antibody titre is useful for demonstrating that a streptococcal infection has taken place in the recent past. A titre of >200 iu/l usually indicates recent infection.

Treatment

- Most mild attacks of scarlet fever and streptococcal tonsillitis respond to treatment with penicillin V 7 mg/kg, 6 hourly, for 10 days.
- In more severe episodes, benzylpenicillin 20–40 mg/kg, 6 hourly, given iv is prescribed.
- Erythromycin may be given where the patient is allergic to penicillin.
- Flucloxacillin is required if a staphylococcal aetiology is suspected.

Prevention

- Exclude patients from work or school during therapy.
- Cases in hospital should be isolated.

Toxic shock syndrome

Causative agent

- *Staph. aureus*–strains that elaborate toxic shock syndrome toxin type I (TSST-I), or, less commonly, enterotoxin B-producing strains.

Epidemiology and pathophysiology

- An epidemic in the USA amongst children focused attention on this syndrome when first described in 1978, although similar diseases were described as long ago as 1927.
- Toxic shock syndrome has a well-recognized association with menstruation, the use of tampons and coincidental vaginal infection with toxigenic *Staph. aureus*.
- 1–17 cases per 100 000 menstruating women. The risk for women under 30 is 3 times higher than for older women. About 6% of cases are fatal.
- It may also follow skin infections, especially in children.
- There is an associated significant morbidity and mortality (2.5%).

Clinical features

- The diagnostic characteristics are acute onset of fever greater than 38.9°C, postural dizziness or documented hypotension and a diffuse or palmar erythroderma which desquamates on recovery.
- Other features include vomiting or diarrhoea, altered consciousness, impaired renal function, thrombocytopenia, cardiopulmonary dysfunction, hyperaemia of the vagina, oropharynx, or conjunctivae, and decreased serum calcium or phosphate.
- These symptoms last for 1–2 weeks.

Differential diagnosis

- This includes 'toxic' scarlet fever and Kawasaki disease.

Diagnosis

- The diagnosis is usually made on clinical grounds.
- Isolation of TSST-I or enterotoxin B-producing *Staph. aureus* from the vagina, tampon or infected skin wound will support the diagnosis.
- There is an accompanying raised white blood cell count, and abnormal liver and renal function tests.
- Any woman with unexplained fever, vomiting and diarrhoea should be asked about her use of tampons.

Treatment

- Supportive therapy includes iv fluids and, occasionally, more aggressive treatment in the intensive care unit.
- Parenteral flucloxacillin (7–14 mg/kg, 6 hourly) for 7–10 days is also required. iv immunoglobulin may also have a role.

Prevention

- Avoid the use of tampons in women who have had a previous attack, although the organism is most probably a contaminant of the tampon rather than any one woman being particularly susceptible.
- All cases should be isolated.

Erythema multiforme (EM), Stevens–Johnson syndrome, toxic epidermal necrolysis and Ritter's disease

Causative agents

Erythema multiforme, Stevens–Johnson syndrome and toxic epidermal necrolysis

- A wide range of causes include herpes simplex, *Mycoplasma pneumoniae* and *S. pyogenes*.
- Drugs are also an important cause, but many cases are 'idiopathic'.

Ritter's syndrome

- *Staph. aureus* (exfoliatin-producing strains).

Epidemiolgy and pathophysiology

- EM and Stevens–Johnson syndrome can be seen at any age.

- Toxic epidermal necrolysis (Lyell's syndrome) is a disease of older children and adults and, most commonly, it is a drug hypersensitivity reaction.
- Ritter's syndrome affects infants almost exclusively.

Incubation period

- Ritter's syndrome occurs 1–2 days after the staphylococcal infection.
- The other rashes are seen 1–14 days after the underlying stimulus is introduced.

Clinical features

- EM, Stevens–Johnson syndrome and toxic epidermal necrolysis (TEN) are regarded as diseases on a spectrum with EM as the mildest and TEN the most severe manifestation.
- Ritter's syndrome (staphylococcal scalded skin syndrome) is a disease due to toxin producing strains of *Staph. aureus* that is very similar in appearance to TEN.
- EM starts as macules, papules and plaques of varying sizes up to 2 cm, that can be seen anywhere on the body. Typical target lesions are found mainly on the extremities and are identified by their central erythematous macule, papule or vesicle, a surrounding area of more normal skin and an outer erythematous ring. Conjunctivitis, mucosal (especially oral) ulceration and fever when additionally found constitutes the Stevens–Johnson syndrome.
- TEN may start as an EM or Stevens–Johnson-like rash, but rapidly progresses to large fluid-filled bullae and areas of sheared superficial skin leaving extensive denuded areas. Conjunctivitis and mucosal ulceration are also extensive. Sheets of stratum corneum can be readily rubbed off underlying layers of epidermis (Nikolsky's sign).
- EM and Stevens–Johnson syndrome usually heal within 1–4 weeks, although the mucosal ulceration may persist for months.
- Complications may include hepatitis, renal failure, cardiac feature, hypoalbuminaemia and secondary bacterial infection of lesions. The mortality is high.
- Ritter's syndrome starts as a spreading erythematous rash in a febrile infant. After 3 days, the body will also be covered with large bullae and areas of denuded skin. Nikolsky's sign will be present.
- Healing is seen in 2–3 weeks.
- Secondary bacterial infection can be a complicating factor.

Differential diagnosis

- EM-like rashes may be seen in Kawasaki disease, autoimmune and vasculitic conditions. Measles and erythema marginatum (rheumatic fever) may also be mistaken for EM.
- TEN and Ritter's syndrome may be mistaken for other bullous lesions, including pemphigus and pemphigoid. The two conditions are separated by the age of the patient, recognized stimuli in the case of TEN, and, possibly, by skin biopsy.

Diagnosis

- EM and Stevens–Johnson syndrome are diagnosed clinically, but the causative agent should, if possible, be identified to prevent recurrence. This may include investigations for herpes simplex and *M. pneumoniae* or the recognition of a causative drug such as a sulphonamide.
- TEN is more commonly linked to drug sensitivity, which should be identified.
- The causative *Staph. aureus* in Ritter's syndrome can be found in the nasopharynx or skin.

Treatment

- The causative agent or drug should be treated and removed as soon as possible. In the case of Ritter's syndrome, this means flucloxacillin 7–14 mg/kg, 6 hourly, for 7–14 days.
- Steroids have a controversial role in the treatment of the diseases of the EM/TEN spectrum. Supportive therapy includes, as required, iv fluids and nutrition and broad-spectrum antibiotics if secondary skin infection is suspected.

Prevention

- Recurrence of the EM/TEN reactions depends on avoiding the causative drugs and early treatment of the related infection.
- *Staph. aureus* causing Ritter's syndrome are infectious and cases should be isolated.

Pertussis

Causative agent

- *Bordetella pertussis*, a Gram-negative coccobacillus.

Epidemiology and pathophysiology

- It is droplet spread, mainly in the colder months.
- The disease mainly occurs in childhood, although adults can be affected.
- 15 305 cases were notified in England and Wales in 1990; 7 deaths occurred during the same period.

Incubation period

- 5–14 days.

Clinical features

- The disease begins with the catarrhal stage: cough, temperature and catarrh, which lasts 7–10 days.
- As the temperature subsides, the typical paroxysmal cough develops; a series of coughs is followed by a characteristic whoop (inspiratory high-pitched noise) or vomiting, or both. During a coughing bout, the face becomes congested and subconjunctival haemorrhage may occur. In between bouts of coughing, the child may appear normal, but may progressively become weaker and exhausted.
- The whole illness may last for up to 3 months. (The Chinese call it the cough of 100 days.)
- One episode of whooping cough usually confers lifelong immunity.
- In infants, who suffer the highest morbidity and mortality, the typical cough may be replaced by prolonged apnoeic episodes.
- Complications include lobar collapse, bronchopneumonia, pneumothorax and surgical emphysema.
- Convulsions may be of the febrile type or follow a period of anoxia accompanying a paroxysm.
- Subconjunctival haemorrhage, ulceration of the frenum of the tongue, hernia, prolapsed rectum and brain damage have also been seen.

Differential diagnosis

- The prodromal illness is similar to other causes of coryza.
- Prolonged cough may be caused by an inhaled foreign body.

Diagnosis

- *Bordetella pertussis* can be cultured on Bordet–Gengou culture medium or charcoal-yeast extract from a nasopharyngeal swab in charcoal transport medium.

- Swabs are more likely to be positive in the first half of the illness and a negative swab does not disprove the diagnosis.
- A striking blood lymphocytosis is often a feature.

Treatment

- Antibiotics do not appear to alter the clinical course once the illness is well established, although erythromycin 7–15 mg/kg, 6 hourly, for 14 days may ameliorate the disease if given during the prodromal (catarrhal) phase.
- Antibiotics are indicated for secondary pneumonia.

Prevention

- The incidence and mortality from whooping cough have declined since the introduction of vaccination.
- From 1 May 1990, primary vaccination has been offered to all infants at the age of 2, 3 and 4 months.
- Pertussis is usually given as part of the triple (diphtheria, pertussis, tetanus) vaccine. Monovalent vaccine is also available.
- Reinforcing doses of vaccine may be considered for household contacts under 7 years old.
- A full course of vaccine confers protection in over 80% of recipients and, in those not fully protected, the course of the disease is much less severe.
- Whooping cough vaccine is a killed vaccine.
- A new acellular vaccine is being researched and is said to cause fewer reactions and possibly a greater immunogenicity.
- Erythromycin prophylaxis (7–15 mg/kg, 6 hourly, for 5 days) may prevent disease in non-immune children who are household contacts.

Mumps

Causative agent

- A large myxovirus.

Epidemiology and pathophysiology

- Infectivity lasts from just before the onset of parotid swelling until the swelling in the glands has completely disappeared and is spread by droplet, kissing or fomites.

- It is mainly a disease of 2–5-year-old children with a peak incidence in late winter and spring.
- There are 1200 hospital admissions per year in England and Wales. In the under 15-year-old age-group, it is the commonest cause of viral meningitis.
- 4271 cases were notified in 1990.

Incubation period

- 14–28 days.

Clinical features

- In one-third of cases, there are no symptoms. A prodromal illness, lasting for 24 hours, of fever, malaise and headache is the first sign of infection. Parotid swelling is the most common manifestation, although the sublingual and submaxillary glands may also be involved. Swellings may be unilateral or bilateral. There is associated fever and pain on swallowing.
- Other symptoms include fever, headaches and vomiting. The illness lasts approximately 7 days.
- Complications include meningitis, encephalitis, deafness, orchitis, oophoritis and pancreatitis. Orchitis does *not* lead to sterility.
- Rarer complications include arthritis, mastitis, nephritis, thyroiditis, pericarditis and pneumonitis.

Differential diagnosis

- Parotid swelling can also be due to pyogenic infection, tumour or sarcoidosis.
- Cervical adenitis and abscess may produce a swelling similar to mumps. This is usually lower in location and more well-defined than mumps parotitis.

Diagnosis

- The parotid swelling of mumps is ill-defined and envelops the angle of the jaw.
- The virus can be isolated from saliva and urine.
- Serology can be useful, and a lymphocytosis is common on blood film.
- A raised serum amylase confirms parotid inflammation.

Treatment

- Symptomatic relief of the painful parotitis is usually necessary.
- Steroids may be useful to relieve painful orchitis.

Prevention

- The MMR vaccine was introduced in October 1988 and replaces the measles monovalent vaccination.
- It is offered to children between the ages of 1 and 2 years.
- MMR may be given to children who have already been vaccinated against measles.
- Human normal immunoglobulin may ameliorate disease in non-immune close contacts of index cases, but it is of low efficacy.

CHAPTER 12

Infective arthritis and osteomyelitis

AS osteomyelitis is uncommon, except within the setting of trauma, it is frequently not considered as a diagnosis in patients with bone pain, particularly that arising in the back. Arthritis, however, is altogether too obvious in most cases and the major difficulty lies in differentiating the reactive, 'inflammatory' and infective types. As some bacteria can rapidly destroy joint tissue, an early diagnosis is essential and only early referral for joint aspiration will achieve this end.

Therapeutic problems are most likely to arise in osteomyelitis, as the penalty for undertreatment is a high rate of relapse and chronicity. As always in medicine, attention to detail, such as the measurement of minimum bacteriocidal concentrations of antibiotics for an organism, will pay dividends.

Acute infectious arthritis

Causative agents

Bacteria

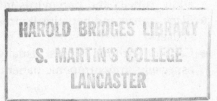

- Staph. aureus.
- S. pneumoniae.
- S. pyogenes.
- Salmonella sp.
- Neisseria gonorrhoeae.
- Enterobacteriaceae.
- Borrelia burgdorferi.
- H. influenzae (in children under 5 years old).
- Mycobacterium tuberculosis.
- A 'reactive' arthritis is seen after many types of gastroenteritis and other bacterial infections including S. pyogenes (rheumatic fever).

Viruses

- Rubella virus.
- Parvovirus B19.
- Hepatitis B virus.
- Mumps virus and others.

Fungi
- *Candida* sp.

Epidemiology and pathophysiology

- With such a wide range of possible causes, epidemiological factors may aid the aetiological diagnosis.
- The disease in young children is most usually a result of haematogenous spread or local invasion through breached skin, in which case *Staph. aureus, S. pyogenes, S. pneumoniae* and *H. influenzae* are important causes.
- In young, sexually active adults, a sexually transmitted organism such as gonorrhoea or non-gonococcal urethritis leading to arthritis as part of Reiter's syndrome (which also includes conjunctivitis, circinate ballanitis and keratoderma blennorrhagica) must be considered.
- If the disease is preceded by diarrhoea then *Salmonella* or another enteric pathogen leading to a secondary 'reactive' arthritis are most likely irrespective of the age of the patient.
- When a polyarthritis forms part of a mild generalized illness, which includes lymphadenopathy and, possibly, a rash in an older child or adult, rubella and parvovirus infection are highly likely.
- *Staph. aureus* and hepatitis B virus are particularly common in iv drug abusers.
- Candida arthritis is most usually the result of infected iv cannulae, especially in neutropenic patients.

Clinical features

- In most cases of pyogenic arthritis, a single joint is involved. The most commonly infected include the knee, hip, ankle, elbow and shoulder.
- Symptoms commence with fever, pain and swelling of the affected joint, which becomes stiff and uncomfortable.
- Multiple joint involvement would suggest a viral aetiology or a reactive arthritis.
- When Mycobacterium TB infection involves the joint, the onset is much slower and less painful.
- Complications include joint damage with permanent limitation of movement, epiphyseal involvement in children leading to bone shortening and septicaemia.

Differential diagnosis

- Joint swelling is also a feature of primary rheumatological conditions such as rheumatoid arthritis and of haemarthrosis following trauma.
- Tenosynovitis (inflammation of the tendon sheath) may be mistaken for arthritis.

Diagnosis

- When multiple joints are involved, a pyogenic arthritis is less likely. If other features suggest the aetiology further, such as conjunctivitis and urethritis or diarrhoea in Reiter's syndrome, or rash and lymphadenopathy in the viral diseases, joint aspiration may be avoided.
- When there is any doubt, synovial fluid should be aspirated using an aseptic technique. The final diagnosis depends on the identification of bacteria by Gram-staining or culture. A neutrophil leucocytosis in the joint fluid is also suggestive, but it may be seen in acute rheumatoid arthritis and gout.
- Microscopy of the synovial fluid using polarized light should be used to identify uric acid or pyrophosphate crystals and therefore eliminate gout or pseudo-gout.
- Blood cultures should also be taken, and a raised white blood cell count will suggest a pyogenic infection.
- If there is associated diarrhoea, cultures of stool should be taken.
- When Reiter's syndrome or *N. gonorrhoeae* are likely, chlamydial or gonococcal swabs should be taken from the urethra or female genital tract.
- Specific viral serology (rubella and parvovirus IgM or hepatitis B surface antigen) will establish these agents as the cause.

Treatment

- Antibiotics are required for confirmed or suspected pyogenic arthritis. If a Gram-stain of synovial fluid fails to suggest the cause, an empirical regimen should be used; cefotaxime 30 mg/kg, 8–12 hourly, and flucloxacillin 15 mg/kg, 6 hourly, both given iv, is a suitable combination. Therapy should be for 2–4 weeks.
- Affected joints should be rested from weight-bearing, although passive movement maintained. Analgesics may also be required.

Prevention

- In most cases, prevention is not possible.

Osteomyelitis

Causative agents

- *Staph. aureus.*
- Enterobacteriaceae.
- *Mycobacterium tuberculosis.*

Epidemiology and pathophysiology

- Infection may be introduced by trauma or there may be local spread of infection to the bone, blood-borne spread, or infection of diseased bone.
- Blood-borne infection of normal bone is seen most frequently in children.
- Infections related to trauma, infected fractures and organism spread from local tissue are the usual causes in patients over 5 years.
- Atherosclerosis and diabetes mellitus are also associated with infection in the elderly.
- Tuberculous osteomyelitis will be most commonly observed in ethnic minorities.
- Salmonella osteomyelitis is most common in sickle-cell disease.

Incubation period

- 1–12 weeks.

Clinical features

- In infection of normal bone, fever, malaise, localized pain, tenderness and, sometimes, swelling are often found. In many patients, localized pain alone is the major presentation. Long bones and vertebrae are the most likely to be involved.
- Apart from the history of trauma or associated infection, the presentation of osteomyelitis in this situation is similar.
- Patients with diabetes and atherosclerosis may have infection of the small bones of the feet and experience localized pain and swelling with only mild fever.
- Tuberculous osteomyelitis can be particularly insidious in onset.
- Untreated infection can become chronic, with sinus formation and associated amyloid disease.

Differential diagnosis

- Soft-tissue infection, fracture and tumours can all be mistaken for osteomyelitis.

Diagnosis

- The typical X-ray changes of bone lucency, followed by cortical irregularities and periosteal expansion, will be seen after 2 weeks. There is usually an associated soft-tissue swelling. In late cases, an intramedullary sequestrum may be seen.
- In difficult cases, a scan utilizing radioactive gallium or technetium may localize such infection.
- The aetiological diagnosis should be established by a combination of blood, bone-aspiration and bone-drainage cultures.
- The white blood cell count and ESR will normally be raised.

Treatment

- Acute osteomyelitis requires therapy for a least 4 weeks using iv antibiotics for at least part of this time. Antibiotic usage will be guided by the sensitivity of identified organisms, but dosage should be adjusted to achieve trough serum levels greater than the *in vitro* minimum bacteriocidal concentration for that organism.
- Chronic osteomyelitis requires antibiotic therapy as above for 3 months or more and, in addition, surgery with débridement of dead bone.
- Tuberculous osteomyelitis requires standard therapy for 2 years and often longer because relapse is common.

Prevention

- Only post-traumatic osteomyelitis is preventable by adequate wound toilet, sterile surgical technique and the use of prophylactic antibiotics.

CHAPTER 13

Human immunodeficiency virus and its complications

DESPITE the large amount of publicity and fear engendered by HIV and AIDS, they remain relatively uncommon conditions outside the few cities in the UK where infected homosexual men and iv drug abusers are concentrated, although heterosexual infection is on the rise. This contrasts with parts of Africa where heterosexual infection is commonplace. Nevertheless, it is important to be aware of these conditions because of their high morbidity and mortality, and the need to avoid accidental infection of medical staff. As with other infectious diseases, the common pattern of disease presentation has been rapidly established and its management in most cases has become a familiar routine. However, the large number of possible secondary infections and malignacies require a wide range of diagnostic and therapeutic skills and facilities.

This chapter is meant to give only a brief entrée to the condition and its many facets. Although only the more common infectious manifestations have been described, this is not to decry the immense social and psychological aspects of this disease.

Human immunodeficiency virus infections

Causative agents

● HIV types 1 and 2. These are retroviruses that utilize the enzyme reverse transcriptase to produce deoxyribonucleic acid (DNA) intermediates from the virus RNA template. The DNA so produced can integrate into the host DNA permanently.

Epidemiology and pathophysiology

● The infection was first recognized in 1981 in homosexual men and Haitian immigrants to the USA, although HIV-1 was first isolated only in 1983.
● Transmission is parenteral or sexual and there are several well-defined risk groups: homosexual men; iv drug abusers; recipients of blood, blood products or body tissues; promiscuous heterosexuals,

especially prostitutes; sexual contacts of the inhabitants of many underdeveloped countries, especially in East Africa; the sexual partner of someone in one of these groups and infants born to females in a risk group. Some infected individuals admit to none of these risk factors.

- Transplacental infection as well as breast milk transmission is possible.
- There were over 3700 cases of AIDS reported in England and Wales, with over 50% dead, by 1990.
- By March 1991 there were 4226 cases of AIDS in the UK:

    3489 in gay men
     140 in drug abusers
      66 in gay drug abusers
     272 related to blood/blood products
      16 vertically transmitted
      48 undetermined
     195 heterosexually transmitted.

Of the latter category only 13 (0.3%) occurred in people whose partner was not in a high risk group (haemophiliac, bisexual, drug abuser, partner from abroad).

These figures show an overall rise in heterosexually transmitted disease (now 18%) although the majority are in people whose partner is in a known 'at risk' group.

- Estimates of HIV infection suggest up to 100 000 cases in England and Wales. A 'gay' life-style and drug abuse accounts for most of the cases at present.
- HIV-2 is a similar virus to HIV-1 in all respects except that it is largely confined to West Africa or people connected with this area and causes less severe disease.

Incubation period

- Seroconversion illness normally occurs 2–6 weeks after exposure with anti-HIV antibody being positive 3–12 weeks after exposure. HIV antigen can be detected transiently 1–4 weeks after infection.

Clinical features

- Symptoms may be due to either HIV itself or other infections and malignancies that arise out of the suppression of T4 (CD4 + ve) helper lymphocytes by this disease.

● The first classification of HIV-related disease, which is still sometimes used, described asymptomatic disease, persistent generalized lymphadenopathy, AIDS-related complex and AIDS. This has several drawbacks, such as the spurious suggestion inherent in this scheme that there is a smooth progession from asymptomatic disease to AIDS. This method remains the main epidemiological tool used for surveillance in the UK.

● Other schemes include the Walter Reed classification, and the Centers for Disease Control (CDC) classification system of HIV infection, which is becoming very popular and will be described in detail.

● **CDC Group I** disease is the acute 'seroconversion' illness, 2–6 weeks after acquisition of the virus a proportion, estimated variously as 10–90%, develop symptoms. These may include fever, lymphadenopathy, generalized rash, sore throat, myalgia, anorexia, diarrhoea and orogenital ulceration. Aseptic meningitis, encephalitis, peripheral neuropathy and Guillain–Barré syndrome may also occur. Most symptoms remit spontaneously in 2–4 weeks.

● **CDC Group II** is asymptomatic infection. A patient may be anti-HIV ('body') positive without symptoms or signs for many years before progressing to Group III or IV disease.

● **CDC Group III** disease is the stage of persistent generalized lymphadenopathy in which enlarged lymph nodes in at least 2 extra-inguinal sites persist for over 3 months. At least 50% of patients exhibit this manifestation.

● **CDC Group IV** includes all of what was previously classified as AIDS related complex (ARC) or AIDS and is seen in a median time of 10 years after primary infection. It is divided into:

   IVA – constitutional disease, such as fatigue, fever, night sweats, diarrhoea and weight loss (known as HIV wasting syndrome);
   IVB – neurological disease, including HIV encephalopathy and peripheral neuropathy.
   IVC$_1$ – the secondary infections categorized in the CDC classification of AIDS. Virus infections include CMV involvement of gut, lung or eyes, severe herpes simplex infection outside the mouth, and progressive multifocal leucoencephalopathy. Bacterial manifestations can be recurrent salmonella septicaemia, disseminated Mycobacterium avium intracellulare complex (MAI), extrapulmonary *M. tuberculosis* and recurrent bacterial infection in HIV-positive children (<13 years old). Protozoal infections seen are cryptosporidia gastroenteritis, cerebral toxoplasmosis, isospora gastroenteritis and pneumocystis pneumonitis. Fungal disease manifests as extrapulmonary cryptococcal infection and severe candidal involvement of the oesophagus, airways or lungs.

IVC$_2$ describes infection not classified as AIDS, such as shingles and oral candidiasis.

IVD includes the secondary cancers associated with HIV: Kaposi's sarcoma, CNS lymphoma, specified non-Hodgkin's lymphoma and other less common malignancies.

IVE is used to describe other conditions related to HIV. Lymphoid interstitial pneumonitis in children less than 13 years old is one example.

- Symptom complexes will be described below in more detail.

Diagnosis

- Diagnosis depends on the identification of anti-HIV antibody or HIV antigen, or both, in serum. HIV antigen may be the only marker in the first 6 weeks after infection.
- Other diseases related to HIV should be identified along appropriate lines.
- Serological markers indicative of a poor prognosis include a low T4 lymphocyte count ($<0.4 \times 10^9/l$) a raised level of β2-microglobulin, a positive HIV antigen and negative anti-ϱ24 antibody in serum.
- Hypergammaglobulinaemia, lymphopenia and thrombocytopenia may also be seen.
- Pre-test counselling is recommended in most cases before blood samples are taken.
- HIV testing is normally carried out after informed consent from the patient, although AIDS can be diagnosed in the absence of a known antibody status when certain associated diseases are recognized.

Treatment

- Antiviral therapy is now usually introduced when the blood T4 count is $<0.4 \times 10^9/l$ irrespective of the symptoms present. Recent evidence suggests a benefit from therapy at higher T4 counts. Zidovudine 250 mg 4 times daily is the only agent of proven benefit, although its effects seems to wane after 6 months due to disease progression and viral resistance. Other promising agents are under trial.
- Prophylactic antibiotics are being increasingly introduced before secondary infections supervene (primary prophylaxis) or after the first attack of superinfection (secondary prophylaxis). Nebulized pentamidine to prevent *Pneumocystis carinii pneumonitis* (PCP) and antifungal agents for candidiasis are examples.
- Most patients require extensive social support and easy access to medical care.
- Treatment should include counselling, education and support.

Prevention

- This can be achieved through sexual monogamy with an uninfected partner, testing of blood and blood products, and the use of sterile needles and syringes by drug addicts.
- Vaccines are being researched.
- Other measures that may be helpful are the practice of safe sex (condoms, oral sex, etc.) and the avoidance of pregnancy in women at risk.
- Needlestick injury and contamination of wounds by the bodily fluids of infected individuals poses a particular problem to health-care workers and it can be prevented by the appropriate use of gloves, eye protection and proper sharps disposal. Zidovudine prophylaxis does not seem to work.
- Avoidance of blood transfusions in countries without donor screening.

Dysphagia in the HIV-positive patient

Causative agents

- *Candida albicans.*
- CMV.
- HSV.

Epidemiology

- Oral disease, especially infection with *Candida* is very common, and oesophageal involvement occurs in 3% of HIV-positive individuals at presentation with AIDS.

Clinical features

- Oral discomfort is most commonly due to *Candida* when creamy, thick plaques can be seen in any part of the buccal cavity. Occasionally, this infection presents as erythematous plaques (atrophic *Candida*). Extensive ulceration due to herpes simplex gingivostomatitis may also be a cause. Less commonly, bacterial gingivitis may be found.
- Retrosternal discomfort, especially on swallowing, with nausea and anorexia, is again most commonly due to *Candida*. Profound weight loss can result. Herpes simplex and CMV can present as a severe ulcerative oesophagitis.

Differential diagnosis

- Oral hairy leucoplakia, white plaques on the oral mucosa caused by infection with EBV may mimic symptoms of infection with *Candida*.
- Gastric CMV and Kaposi's sarcoma may cause similar symptoms and will be diagnosed on gastroscopy.

Diagnosis

- Oral infection with *Candida* is usually clinically obvious, but it can be confirmed by culture of swabs. If dysphagia is also present, this is most often due to candidal oesophagitis.
- Other causes of oral disease can be confirmed by appropriate viral and bacterial swabs or, less commonly, by biopsy.
- In most cases of oesophagitis when infection with *Candida* is suspected, a therapeutic trial of antifungal therapy may be tried. If a firm diagnosis is essential, or infection with *Candida* is excluded, oesophagoscopic biopsy and viral culture is indicated.

Treatment

- Oral infection with *Candida* responds to local nystatin or amphotericin, whereas more extensive disease is best treated with systemic agents such as ketoconazole or the safer fluconazole. Therapy on full dosage is continued until resolution of symptoms following which prophylactic doses may be given indefinitely.
- Herpes simplex infection is treated with oral acyclovir (200 mg 5 times daily) until at least 2 days after resolution. Prophylaxis may be considered in some patients.
- CMV infection will respond to ganciclovir 5 mg/kg, 12 hourly, iv, but response is often poor or incomplete. More recently, forscarnet has been used with success. Prophylactic therapy is most usually required.

Prevention

- Some doctors are prescribing acyclovir and antifungal agents (e.g. fluconazole) as primary prophylaxis.

Liver disease in HIV infection

Causative agents

- Hepatitis A,B,C and D viruses.
- CMV.

- EBV.
- MAI.
- *Mycobacterium tuberculosis*.
- *Cryptosporidium parvum*.
- Drugs, alcohol and Kaposi's sarcoma.

Epidemiology

- HIV-positive patients acquire the infection by the same route as many of the hepatitis-related viruses, consequently the two commonly co-exist.
- Drug reactions are very common in HIV-infected patients.

Clinical features

- Many patients will already have chronic liver disease due to hepatitis B, which is usually mild as HIV infection ameliorates the symptoms. Hepatitis C and D tend to get worse in this situation and may present as developing jaundice or decompensating liver disease.
- Right hypochondrial discomfort, jaundice and hepatomegaly can have a variety of causes. When fever is also a feature, infection with MAI, *Mycobacterium tuberculosis*, or drug reaction should be suspected. This process may progress to liver failure.

Diagnosis

- The pattern of LFTs may suggest the cause, with a high aminotransferase level (hepatocellular) being associated with virus infections in particular. A raised alkaline phosphatase (obstructive) pattern might suggest drugs (e.g. sulphonamides), cholangitis due to cryptosporidia or the mycobacterial infections. These associations are not entirely specific and there is much crossover between the causes and their effects.
- Blood culture, serology and biopsy of other affected sites may indicate the cause, as may liver and biliary tract imaging.
- In many cases, a liver biopsy is required to identify the cause, utilizing histology and bacterial and viral culture.

Treatment

- Withdrawal of suspected drugs or alcohol may lead to improvement. The viral causes are more difficult to deal with as is infection with cryptosporidia, although some success has been achieved with alpha-interferon in infection with the hepatotropic viruses.

- Infection with *Mycobacterium tuberculosis* responds adequately to conventional antibiotics (*see* section on TB, page 41), whereas that with MAI responds very poorly.

Prevention

- Hepatitis B vaccine may be offered to patients with early HIV infection and an intact immune system.

Diarrhoea in HIV infection

Causative agents

- All causes listed in Chapter 6 on gastrointestinal infection may be found in patients with HIV infection.
- *Cryptosporidium parvum*, *Isospora belli*, microsporidia, CMV, adenovirus, Giardia and MAI are particularly common.
- Kaposi's sarcoma and lymphoma.

Epidemiology

- HIV infection *per se* may be implicated as a part of the HIV wasting syndrome.
- Diarrhoea is particularly common in late HIV infection.

Clinical features

- Diarrhoea, which may be accompanied by fever, abdominal pain, vomiting and bloating, can have a variety of causes.
- *Cryptosporidium parvum* is particularly associated with prolonged watery diarrhoea and weight loss.
- Salmonella infection may cause recurrent septicaemia and is one of the diagnostic criteria for AIDS.

Diagnosis

- Culture of stool for bacteria, microscopy of stool and rectal biopsy taken for microscopy and viral culture will identify the pathogen in up to 85% of diarrhoeal episodes.

Treatment

- Pathogens identified as a cause of diarrhoea are more likely to require antimicrobial therapy in HIV positive patients than in immunocompetent patients.

- Salmonella infection requires ciprofloxacin 7–10 mg/kg, 12 hourly, orally, especially if *Salmonella* is detected on blood cultures. Prolonged therapy is frequently required.
- Cryptosporidial enteritis does not respond to antimicrobials, and treatment centres around fluid and electrolyte replacement and the use of antidiarrhoeal agents such as loperamide.

Prevention

- Many of these agents are transmissible and afflicted patients should be isolated.

Lung disease in HIV infection

Causative agents

- *Pneumocystis carinii.*
- *Mycobacterium tuberculosis.*
- MAI.
- *Cryptococcus neoformans.*
- CMV.
- All causes of pneumonia listed in that section can be found in this setting; recurrent bacterial infection is particulary common in infected children.

Epidemiology

- PCP is seen in at least 65% of AIDS patients.
- Lung infection is one of the commonest manifestations of CDC Group IV disease.
- Multiple infection is common.

Clinical features

- PCP may cause a wide range of symptoms varying from prolonged lethargy without fever, through acute pneumonitis with cough, dyspnoea and fever to fulminant respiratory failure. The mortality rate is 20–25%.
- Other pathogens may have a similar presentation, although bacterial infections are more likely to be associated with productive cough.
- Physical findings usually include dyspnoea and tachypnoea (particularly noticeable after minimal exertion), and may also include signs of consolidation, such as inspiratory crackles and bronchial breathing.

Diagnosis

- An initial chest X-ray can be helpful in deciding the aetiology. A pleural effusion suggests a bacterial or malignant cause. Hilar adenopathy is most likely to be associated with a malignancy or mycobacterial infection. The different organisms can cause a variety of changes within the lung fields. A normal chest X-ray can be found in PCP or cryptococcal infection.
- For PCP, therapy is instituted usually whilst further investigations are being carried out. Hypoxaemia, worsened by exercise, suggests a diffuse pneumonitis, such as that seen with PCP or CMV infection. Sputum, induced by inhalation of nebulized saline, may allow identification of the pathogen when examined microscopically and cultured for bacteria, viruses and fungi.
- When the diagnosis remains unclear and response to empirical therapy for PCP is slow, bronchoscopy and broncho-alveolar lavage will usually confirm the aetiological diagnosis.

Treatment

- If PCP seems likely, therapy with co-trimoxazole (20 mg/kg trimethoprim and 100 mg/kg sulphamethoxazole) in 2 or more divided doses daily for 2–3 weeks will be effective. Drug-induced fever, rash, jaundice and marrow suppression are common. In milder cases, nebulized pentamidine 600 mg daily for 3 weeks is useful. Alternative agents include iv pentamidine, trimetrexate, pyrimethamine/dapsone and pyrimethamine/sulphadiazine. Oxygen, steroids and, less commonly, assisted ventilation may also be required. Treatment failures are relatively common.
- CMV is often found, but it is not necessarily a serious pathogen and, in any case, it responds very poorly to therapy.
- MAI also responds poorly whereas *Mycobacterium tuberculosis* can be eradicated by conventional antituberculosis therapy.

Prevention

- Primary prophylaxis for PCP (with daily co-trimoxazole or fortnightly nebulized pentamidine) and TB (with daily isoniazid) have been recommended by some for patients with a T4 count $<0.4 \times 10^9/l$. Secondary prophylaxis is usually instituted after cure.

Infection of the central nervous system in HIV infection

Causative agents

● Papovavirus (JC virus).
● CMV.
● *Toxoplasma gondii.*
● *Cryptococcus neoformans.*
● *Mycobacterium* spp.

Epidemiology

● Some degree of HIV encephalopathy can be found in up to 75% of AIDS patients.
● Cerebral toxoplasmosis occurs in approximately 2% and cryptococcal meningitis in 10% of AIDS patients.

Clinical features

● There are 3 CNS syndromes; meningitis, dementia/encephalopathy and mass lesions.
● Aseptic meningitis can be seen early and is most often due to HIV infection alone. Headache, fever, nausea, vomiting and some neck stiffness may be seen. In late stage disease, *Cryptococcus neoformans* is the major pathogen and presents with fever, malaise and headache, without necessarily being accompanied by other classic features of meningitis. This disease may progress to multisystem involvement with a poorer prognosis. In African patients, TB meningitis should be considered.
● HIV encephalopathy can be found to some degree in 75% of patients with Group IV disease, mainly manifest as an impairment of memory and inability to think quickly. This less commonly progresses to major cognitive dysfunction, seizures, coma and death.
● A similar picture, usually associated with headaches and focal neurological signs, including ataxia and unilateral weakness, may be caused by JC virus in progressive multifocal leucoencephalopathy (PML). Death normally results in less than 3 months.
● Intracerebral mass lesions often present with headache, ataxia, focal weakness or fits. Fever may also be a feature but, as with other HIV-related illness, the signs can be very subtle. Toxoplasmosis is the commonest cause of this syndrome (although it may also present as a diffuse encephalopathy); lymphoma, PML and mycobacterial infections should also be considered.

- The retinopathy due to CMV is best considered here. Progressive visual deterioration is the most common symptom, often starting in one eye. Untreated, retinal detachment and blindness may rapidly supervene. Ophthalmoscopic examination of the retina reveals white exudates, often surrounded by oedema and haemorrhage.

Diagnosis

- Lumbar puncture in patients with HIV meningitis and meningitis due to *Cryptococcus* usually reveals a lymphocytic reaction, slightly raised protein and normal glucose. India-ink stain or electrophoresis for cryptococcal antigens will confirm the latter diagnosis. Some cases of cryptococcal meningitis (approximately 40%) are associated with a normal CSF cell count.
- The CSF is usually normal in HIV encephalopathy, although a raised protein, especially immunoglobulins, may be a feature. CT scanning and EEG show non-specific changes such that this diagnosis is mainly clinical before death. PML is best diagnosed by CT scanning when multiple low density areas are seen in the white matter.
- CT screening is also the most helpful investigation for identifying mass lesions. Those due to *Toxoplasma gondii* are multiple and show ring enhancement after injection of contrast medium. Most patients will also have a positive toxoplasma antibody test, although often in low titre. Less commonly, brain biopsy is required if infection with *Toxoplasma* seems unlikely.
- Confirmation of CMV retinitis may be attained by the finding of virus in blood or urine.

Treatment

- HIV meningitis is usually self-limiting. The encephalopathy may initially respond to zidovudine therapy given on a long-term basis. Relapse is common. PML is untreatable at present.
- *Cryptococcus neoformans* infection is best treated with iv amphotericin B 0.5–1.5 mg/kg daily. The dose must be slowly built up and may require concurrent antihistamines or steroids. A central venous access is required. Treatment for several weeks is required, followed by regular prophylactic doses for the long term. Flucytosine is often given concurrently although recent work suggests a lack of synergy. Fluconazole may also work (200–400 mg daily) and has the advantage that prophylaxis given by the oral route may subsequently be effective.

- Toxoplasmosis will usually respond to pyrimethamine and sulpha-diazine, although the latter may be replaced by clindamycin if severe reactions supervene. A response is normally seen within a week, although treatment is usually continued for 4 weeks until CT scanning and clinical evidence suggest no further response.
- CMV retinitis requires ganciclovir or foscarnet, as described previously.

Prevention

- HIV encephalopathy may be falling in incidence as zidovudine is now given routinely to patients before CDC Group IV disease is manifest.
- Oral fluconazole given as prophylaxis for candidal infection may also reduce the incidence of cryptococcal infection. After cryptococcal disease has become manifest, secondary prophylaxis with amphotericin or fluconazole is invariably required.
- Relapse of toxoplasmosis is common unless regular prophylaxis with drugs, such as Fansidar, is given.
- Ganciclovir or foscarnet should be continued intermittently and indefinitely after CMV retinitis.

Other disease in HIV infection

Causative agents

- MAI.
- *Mycobacterium tuberculosis.*
- CMV.
- *Cryptococcus neoformans.*
- Other invasive fungi.
- Kaposi's sarcoma, lymphoma, other malignancies.

Epidemiology

- African patients with AIDS (CDC Group IV disease) most commonly present with TB or HIV wasting syndrome.
- In the USA, invasive fungal infections should be considered as a cause of pneumonitis or fever.

Clinical features

- A non-specific presentation with fever alone is common and several possibilities should be considered. PCP is a very common cause, as is disseminated CMV, infection with *Cryptococcus neoformans*, mycobacterial disease and, in the immigrant, a systemic fungal infection such as histoplasmosis.
- Many of these diseases cause lymphadenopathy, which may be mistaken for persistent generalized lymphadenopathy. Lymphoma and other disseminated malignancies including Kaposi's sarcoma should also be considered.
- Kaposi's sarcoma is a common manifestation of HIV infection, presenting as skin lesions which are most often red or purple, nodules or plaques.

Diagnosis

- In the undiagnosed febrile patient, consideration should be given to the conditions previously described. PCP must be sought in the Caucasian and TB in the African. Blood cultures including inoculation of special media for MAI and CMV should be routinely used. The latter should be sought in the urine. Chest X-ray is mandatory and lymph-node biopsy can also be helpful.

Treatment

- This is as described previously.
- Systemic fungal infections are treated with amphotericin B. Lymphomas may respond to radiotherapy or cytotoxic drugs. Kaposi's sarcoma has also been treated in this way although patients with a high T4 count may respond to alpha-interferon.

Prevention

- Primary prophylaxis with isoniazid has been suggested for patients who are Mantoux-positive although this is probably impractical.

CHAPTER 14

Infection in the traveller

WITH increasing affluence, decreasing costs of travel and more leisure time, there is a continuing rise in the numbers of people visiting the tropics and subtropics. Added to these are the large numbers of UK residents returning for holiday visits to their former country of residence, and new visitors from the tropics. There is, therefore, a large and rising number of people at risk from tropical infections.

The purpose of this chapter is to emphasize the important and more commonly imported infections and their management.

Despite the recent high profile given to the subject, there is still an unacceptable number of deaths due to malaria and illness related to other serious imported infections because the doctor fails to ask the question: 'where have you been?'. Even when the patient draws attention to their recent foreign travel, some doctors have mistakenly dismissed the diagnosis of malaria or typhoid because of their misconceptions about these diseases. Early investigation and advice from experts should be the rule in the management of febrile travellers. Multiple infections including gut parasites are common.

Appropriate vaccination and information on hygiene will greatly help the intending traveller to avoid illness. It therefore behoves the doctor to keep up to date with the changing situation relating to tropical diseases and to use judiciously the services of specialist vaccination clinics.

Management of the febrile traveller

Causative agents

- *Plasmodium falciparum* and other malarial parasites.
- *Salmonella typhi* and *paratyphi*.
- *Mycobacterium tuberculosis*
- Viral haemorrhagic fevers (Lassa, Ebola, Marburg and Congo–Crimea haemorrhagic fevers).
- HIV.
- *Rickettsia* spp. (typhus).
- *Entamoeba histolytica*.
- *Leptospira* spp.
- *Brucella* spp.

Clinical features

- Although there is a wide range of possible causes of fever, in practice there are only a few that are important.
- Lassa fever has a non-specific onset, often with upper respiratory symptoms and is difficult to recognize clinically.
- Plasmodium falciparum fever is continuous and swinging in most cases; the textbook tertian pattern is extremely rare. A wide range of additional symptoms including diarrhoea, jaundice and cough may be found. A swinging fever is also the only consistent feature of typhoid. Both diseases have a high morbidity and mortality.
- Extrapulmonary TB is particularly common in Asian patients and children in whom fever may be the only symptom. Temperatures up to 40°C with rigors are frequently found. Failure to establish this diagnosis at an early stage may allow progression to tuberculous meningitis.
- Despite the descriptions found in many textbooks, typhus frequently produces a febrile illness without a generalized rash or eschar. There are many geographical variations, but African tick typhus (*R. connorii*) imported from East and Southern Africa is most likely to be encountered.
- Although *Entamoeba histolytica* most frequently presents as a diarrhoeal illness, young male visitors to the tropics are especially at risk of acquiring an amoebic liver abscess. Diarrhoea is found in less than 50% and right hypochondrial pain is frequently mild or absent initially.
- Brucellosis is still endemic wherever pasteurization of milk and cheese is not performed. This disease is a classic cause of non-specific febrile illness which may be prolonged.

Differential diagnosis

- If Lassa fever is likely, the patient will be removed by appropriate ambulance to a designated centre experienced in the investigation of such patients.
- All other febrile patients, no matter how well, should be referred to a centre with experience in the management of infections and tropical diseases for multiple blood film examination and in-patient investigation with blood cultures if necessary. Malaria and typhoid can then be diagnosed early and treated optimally.
- Lumbar puncture or liver biopsy should be considered for the ill child or immigrant in whom there is no evidence of the other conditions, in order to establish a diagnosis of disseminated TB.

- HIV testing should be considered in those with a history of risk, particularly, in this context, sexual contacts of residents of East Africa, Southern Africa, parts of South East Asia and some regions of South America, especially Brazil.
- Typhus is essentially a clinical diagnosis because antibody testing is insensitive and only able to confirm the presence of infection retrospectively.
- Leptospirosis and brucellosis are also most commonly diagnosed serologically, although both of these organisms may be isolated from body fluids.
- Amoebic liver abscess is established by ultrasound imaging of the liver and an antibody test. Aspiration of the abscess may allow identification of trophozoites in the pus.

Diagnosis

- The investigation of the febrile traveller relies first of all on a detailed travel history including information on rural, sexual, water and dietary exposure.
- Antimalarial prophylaxis and immunizations, even when given under ideal circumstances, may still fail, and should *not* be used as a reason to exclude any diagnosis, especially of malaria and typhoid.
- A history of travel outside of the major cities in West and Central Africa in a febrile patient should raise the suspicion of Lassa fever and expert advice from the local CCDC, one of the High Security Isolation Units, and the Communicable Disease Surveillance Centre (081 200 6868), or Communicable Disease (Scotland) (041 946 7120) should be sought.
- In the patient returned from West or Central Africa within 3 weeks of the onset of fever, Lassa fever should be considered.
- Malaria and typhoid should be considered in all patients *irrespective* of accompanying symptoms.
- HIV as a cause of fever in its own right, or associated with other 'tropical' conditions, is an increasing problem in immigrants and long-term visitors who have arrived from East Africa and other tropical countries. A history of sexual contact should be sought, and other STDs, including syphilis, excluded.
- Leptospirosis (*see* Chapter 6) is a relatively common disease in the tropics and should always be considered in any febrile patients. Several cases were recently imported among holiday makers rafting in Northern Thailand.
- Typhoid and paratyphoid will be cultured from blood or stool unless antibiotics have been given previously.

Treatment

- Malaria will be identified by an experienced observer examining several blood films. 'Film-negative' malaria is exceptionally rare.
- Speculative therapy with antibiotics or antimalarials often creates more problems than it solves. Quinine therapy given to a patient 'just in case' he/she has malaria is unjustified; if parasites are found, therapy is given as outlined in the section on malaria (page 162).
- Chloramphenicol (15 mg/kg, 8 hourly) or ciprofloxacin 7 mg/kg, 12 hourly, both orally, will effectively treat typhoid and paratyphoid and may be considered as therapy before confirmation of the diagnosis only if the patient is seriously ill.
- Therapy for the other conditions is outlined elsewhere.
- In the seriously ill patient in whom therapy must be initiated before the diagnosis can be confirmed, those with hypotension, for instance, parenteral quinine and chloramphenicol or ciprofloxacin (in adults only) may be useful.

Prevention

- Typhoid is reduced in incidence by vaccination and antimalarials will prevent most cases of malaria.
- Many of the other conditions can be prevented by good hygiene.

Diarrhoea in the traveller

Causative agents

- All the causes listed in Chapter 6 should be considered, but especially: *Shigella dyseneteriae, Shigella boydii, Shigella flexneri, Vibrio cholerae, Salmonella paratyphi, Giardia lamblia, Entamoeba histolytica* and ETEC.
- Plasmodium falciparum malaria can cause severe diarrhoea.

Epidemiology

- Diarrhoea is probably the commonest cause of ill health in visitors abroad; in one recent survey, 28% of those interviewed said they had suffered.
- These diseases are acquired in contaminated food or water. The warmer climate in the tropics and subtropics encourages the multiplication of pathogenic organisms within food.

Clinical features

- A large proportion of travellers to less developed countries will suffer watery diarrhoea lasting 1–7 days, starting within 3 weeks of arrival. This is almost invariably due to ETEC. It is self-limiting and associated with only a mild fever, although some people may become dehydrated.
- Bacillary dysentery due to the more pathogenic shigellae will present with fever up to 40°C, and diarrhoea that is usually blood-stained. Amoebic dysentery is similar, although the fever is not usually as pronounced. *Campylobacter* and *Salmonella* can also cause such symptoms.
- Paratyphoid especially due to *Salmonella paratyphi* often produces a diarrhoeal illness with a high fever. The stool is green, watery and malodorous. Occasionally, in later stage disease, blood may be present.
- Giardiasis is very common in long-term travellers to the tropics and subtropics. Although vomiting is sometimes a feature of initial disease, the major symptoms include profuse, prolonged water malodorous stool, and marked gas production causing anal and oral flatus ('eggy burps') and borborygmi. Weight loss is often profound.
- Cholera is rare in westerners visiting the tropics because of the association of this disease with grossly contaminated water. Symptoms usually include profuse water ('rice water') stool with little or no fever and vomiting. Profound dehydration, hypotension and death can result.

Differential diagnosis

- When symptoms are more prolonged, two other conditions should be considered: tropical sprue and postinfective irritable bowel syndrome. Tropical sprue is found mainly in travellers who have made prolonged visits especially to India, in whom it causes bulky, offensive, fatty stools and weight loss. Anaemia due to iron and vitamin deficiency may supervene. Postinfective irritable bowel syndrome is a common consequence of travel. There is no weight loss and diarrhoea lasting 1–7 days alternates with normal or constipated stool.
- Coeliac disease and inflammatory bowel disease are sometimes unmasked by the stress of travel and bowel pathogens.

Diagnosis

- Blood cultures are necessary in the febrile patient to identify salmonella bacteraemia. Blood films to exclude falciparum malaria are also mandatory.

- Stool culture will identify the bacterial causes, although special media for vibrios must be used if cholera is to be identified.
- If blood-stained diarrhoea (dysentery) is the problem, microscopy of the stool is helpful. Large numbers of neutrophils in the stool suggest a bacterial aetiology whereas amoeba may be inferred if the neutrophil count is low. Amoebic trophozoites can sometimes be seen in the stool, although a scrape of mucus from the ulcerated rectal mucosa is more likely to allow their identification.
- Stool microscopy after a concentration method will identify giardia cysts.

Treatment

- The majority of cases respond to rehydration as described previously (Chapter 6).
- When bacillary dysentery is confirmed or highly likely, therapy with ciprofloxacin 500 mg, 12 hourly, by mouth in adults or mecillinam 7–15 mg/kg, 6 hourly, in children for at least 5 days in both groups is effective.
- Amoebic dysentery responds to oral metronidazole 12 mg/kg, 5 hourly, or tinidazole 30 mg/kg daily for 5–10 days is effective.
- *Giardia lamblia* is eradicated by tinidazole 30 mg/kg as a single dose or metronidazole 3 mg/kg, 8 hourly, for 7 days.
- Tetracycline 7 mg/kg, 6 hourly, is effective at reducing the diarrhoea in cholera.

Prevention

- Most episodes can be prevented by adequate food and water hygiene. This includes boiling all water to be drunk and otherwise only drinking bottled (sealed) drinks or pasteurized milk. Filtration and the use of iodine and chlorine added to water are useful measures, but they are not 100% effective.
- Food should be cooked to high temperatures. Salads can be eaten only if home-grown, but soaking in chlorinated water can reduce contamination. Uncooked food is safe only if it can be peeled, as with most fruit.
- There is evidence that prophylactic antibiotics or bismuth salts will prevent ETEC, but this is not generally advised because of the risk of antibiotic resistance arising.
- The cholera vaccine is generally agreed to have little or no efficacy.

Enteric fever

Causative agents

- *Salmonella typhi.*
- *Salmonella paratyphi* A, B or C.
- Occasionally, other salmonellae

Epidemiology and pathophysiology

- Worldwide distribution.
- 10% of cases have not travelled abroad.
- Enteric fever caused by *Salmonella typhi* and *Salmonella paratyphi*, which are only found in man, are acquired from humans, contaminated water or food.
- These organisms may also be transmitted by contaminated milk, shellfish or other food contaminated by sewage.
- Other salmonellae are mainly food spread (*see* Chapter 6).
- About 300 cases of infection with *Salmonella typhi* per year, and 100 with *Salmonella paratyphi*, A and B, are reported in the UK, with over 80% imported.

Incubation period

- 7–21 days.

Clinical features

- Symptoms may vary greatly, including no symptoms at all.
- Typhoid fever classically presents with a rising temperature, although the pulse rate often does not rise commensurately. Constipation is usual initially, although after a week or so some patients develop diarrhoea. The patient is often ill and weak. Extremely sparse erythematous macules ('Rose spots') occur in up to 45% of light-skinned patients on about the 10th day, usually involving the abdomen, flanks or chest. A dry cough (typhoidal bronchitis) is common. The illness may last for 3–4 weeks before recovery, unless major complications (see below) occur.
- In addition to a temperature up to 40°C and slow ponderous speech, splenomegaly can be found in 25–65%.
- Complications may include multiple small bowel perforations leading to peritonitis, and gastrointestinal haemorrhage.
- Hepatitis and severe depression are also commonly found.

● Chronic carriage in a diseased gallbladder or kidney allows prolonged gut or urinary excretion.

Differential diagnosis

● See 'Management of the febrile traveller', page 154.

Diagnosis

● Blood culture is most commonly positive in the first week after which the yield falls. Three sets are required for optimal identification.
● Identification of the organism from the faeces is usually more successful after the first week.
● Marrow culture can be successful if other sources fail, especially if antibiotics have been administered.
● The Widal test for salmonella antibodies is unhelpful.

Treatment

● Although amoxycillin, trimethoprim and mecillinam can be effective, the drugs of choice are chloramphenicol 15 mg/kg, 8 hourly, or ciprofloxacin 7 mg/kg, 12 hourly, both given orally for up to 14 days.
● Relapse is common (up to 10%); it can be treated with the same antibiotic as that used in the primary attack.
● Chronic carriage may be eradicated by ciprofloxacin given as above.
● Patients may be isolated until up to 6 consecutive stool cultures *post* treatment are negative.
● Perforation of the gut is usually treated surgically, although medical therapy alone can be successful.

Prevention

● Maintaining adequate standards of hygiene (*see* section on diarrhoea, page 52).
● The typhoid vaccine is effective in reducing the attack rate by about 85%.
● Food handlers are usually debarred from work until the stool culture is consistently negative.
● Liaison with the local CCDC is imperative and all new cases should be notified by telephone.

Malaria

Causative agents

- *Plasmodium falciparum.*
- *Plasmodium vivax.*
- *Plasmodium malariae.*
- *Plasmodium ovale.*

Epidemiology and pathophysiology

- These infections are widespread throughout the tropics and subtropics. Occasional cases have been seen in temperate countries in people living close to airports after accidental importation of infected mosquitoes.
- Anopheline mosquitoes transmit the infection when the female takes a blood meal.
- Other routes include blood and marrow transfusions and transplacental spread.
- The majority of cases reported in the UK are from subsaharan Africa (mainly *Plasmodium falciparum*) and India (mainly *Plasmodium vivax*). For travellers from the UK the greatest risk is from West Africa, where 2% of people who visit Ghana will return with infection due to *Plasmodium falciparum.*
- In 1988, there were 1600 reported cases in England and Wales, 1000 of which were due to *Plasmodium falciparum.* In 1990 there were 1505 cases reported in England and Wales, with 4 deaths. Estimates of global infection suggest up to 200 million cases and 1 million deaths (in Africa) each year.
- There were 7 deaths in England and Wales in 1988 and 1989, all of which were due to infection with *Plasmodium falciparum.*

Incubation period

- This can be as short as 9 days in falciparum malaria, but factors such as antimalarial prophylaxis and partial immunity can delay recognition for up to 1 year for falciparum malaria, 5 years for ovale and vivax malaria and up to 40 years for malariae malaria (in the last 3 cases, it is due to relapse or recrudescence).

Clinical features

- The only typical feature of malaria is fever, which can be as high as 41°C. Almost any other symptom has at one time been associated with malaria, which relects the multisystem involvement of this infection. There is no typical fever pattern in falciparum malaria, although a continuously high swinging fever is the rule, in opposition to the older description of it being a 'malignant tertian' malaria.

● Although the initial fever of the other types is irregular, a typical fever pattern is most likely to develop, This can be tertian (alternate days) in ovale or vivax or quartan (every third day) with malariae malaria.

● Other common symptoms include rigors, headache, nausea and vomiting, myalgia and sweating. Cough and diarrhoea are also frequently experienced.

● Examination may reveal anaemia, jaundice, splenomegaly or hepatomegaly, although none of these features are reliable.

● The 'benign' malarias are so-called because they rarely cause death; untreated attacks eventually peter out. Nonetheless, *Plasmodium malariae* is the commonest cause of nephrotic syndrome in Africa, and the spontaneous or traumatic rupture of an enlarged spleen is often fatal. The 3 non-falciparum malarias have a particular propensity to reappear months or years after exposure due to relapse of a chronic liver stage in the cases of *Plasmodium ovale* and *Plasmodium vivax* or recrudescence of chronic blood carriage with malariae infection.

● Most complications of falciparum malaria are serious, carrying a high mortality rate, especially in the non-immune, although not even those who have lived in endemic areas for all their life achieve more than partial immunity. The major syndromes include cerebral malaria (coma, fits, decerebrate posturing), black water fever (profound haemolysis, haemoglobinuria and renal failure), algid malaria (hypotension, often accompanied by diarrhoea and Gram-negative septicaemia), jaundice (due to haemolysis or malaria hepatitis), acute renal failure, pneumonitis and disseminated intravascular coagulation. Tropical splenomegaly syndrome, an association of massively enlarged spleen, pancytopenia and hyperglobulinaemia is seen in residents of malarious areas and is also thought to be due to *Plasmodium falciparum*.

Differential diagnosis

● This is wide (*see* 'Management of the febrile traveller', page 154) and the most common mistake is to assume that any one feature, or lack of a particular symptom, excludes malaria.

Diagnosis

● Fever in the traveller should be diagnosed as malaria until it is proven otherwise.

- Confirmation is established by the examination of appropriately stained thick and thin films, usually made from a sample taken into an ethylenediaminetetra-acetic acid (EDTA) bottle. Several samples taken at intervals of a few hours may be required to establish the diagnosis. A single sample is *not* enough. 'Slide-negative' malaria is rare and most commonly due to an inexperienced observer having examined the slides.
- In making the diagnosis of malaria do not forget that other infections may co-exist, check the stool for ova cysts and parasites.

Treatment

- Patients with malaria should be treated as in-patients at an experienced unit.
- *Falciparum* malaria is to some degree resistant to chloroquine in virtually all endemic areas. Quinine is the drug of choice. i.v. administration 10 mg/kg up to a maximum of 600 mg over 4 hours every 12 hours (African strains) or every 8 hours (some South East Asian strains) is given for complicated malaria, e.g. cerebral malaria or algid malaria, high parasitaemia (>2–5%) and infection associated with severe vomiting or diarrhoea. Parenteral administration is particularly associated with hypoglycaemia which should be sought routinely and given especial consideration in the drowsy or comatose patient. Dosage reduction may be required in severe infection, especially that associated with hepatic dysfunction, because the drug is metabolized ($>90\%$) mainly in the liver.
- Oral quinine 10 mg/kg up to 600 mg, 8 hourly, is given for uncomplicated attacks and a low parasitaemia and also to the severely ill patient after the parasitaemia has fallen to low levels and recovery is occurring (usually after 1–3 days). Most commonly, 5 days' therapy is followed by Fansidar 3 tablets (in the adult) as a single dose. Other regimens include longer or shorter quinine courses and alternative drugs to Fansidar including mefloquine and tetracycline.
- Complications require appropriate supportive therapies which may be administered in the intensive care or renal units. There has been a vogue for exchange transfusion in patients with very high parasitaemias ($>10\%$ with complications or $>30\%$ without complications), but this form of treatment has not been shown as yet to be a better alternative to optimal medical care.
- Cerebral malaria can occur during therapy, but hypoglycaemia is more common as a cause of deterioration in the level of consciousness.
- Vivax and ovale infections will respond to chloroquine 600 mg stat., 300 mg after 6 hours and 300 mg daily for 2 days. For children aged 1–4, 5–8, and 9–12 years, give ¼, ½ and ¾ of the adult dose,

respectively. Providing the serum glucose-6-phosphate dehydrogenase is normal, primaquine 15 mg daily or 0.2–0.3 mg/kg in children is given by mouth for 14 days to prevent relapse.
- Malaria due to *Plasmodium malariae* responds to chloroquine as above; primaquine is not required.

Prevention

- The attack rate can be reduced by a combination of equally important means.
1 Avoid being bitten. Stay indoors around dawn or dusk, but if outside wear thick, full-length clothing. Use insect repellant, such as diethyltoluamide (DEET), when out of doors. Vapourize pyrethrum through a burning coil (mosquito coil) or heated pad indoors. Air-conditioned rooms also deter mosquitoes, but always have mosquito mesh on windows and doors anyway. Sleep under a mosquito net that is regularly inspected for tears and regularly treated with insect repellant.
2 Antimalarial drugs are also advised. As advice changes regularly, seek up-to-date information before prescribing for travellers. Fansidar and mefloquine are no longer recommended routinely as prophylaxis.

Dengue fever

Causative agents

- Dengue virus serotypes 1–4.
- A flavivirus (RNA).

Epidemiology and pathophysiology

- Dengue fever is found in much of Asia, the Americas and the Caribbean, the Pacific islands and Africa.
- One attack confers immunity for about 9 months, and several episodes will ultimately confer lifelong immunity.
- Some cross-immunity possibly exists between dengue and other flaviviruses, e.g. yellow fever.
- Dengue haemorrhagic fever (DHF) is mainly a disease of school-age children who live in endemic areas.
- It is transmitted by mosquitoes of the genus *Aedes*.
- Incidence increasing in UK, 100 cases reported in 1990.

Incubation period

- 5–9 days.

Clinical features

- Malaise, headache, fever, rigors, retro-orbital, joint and muscle pain are the main symptoms. The temperature may remain elevated for several days and then subside, to be followed by a further period of symptoms and fever – saddle-back fever.
- A discrete maculopapular rash may appear on the 5th to 7th day, often at the time of the second fever. Lymphadenopathy and splenomegaly may be found.
- The major complication is a haemorrhagic state, DHF, which has a mortality rate of approximately 5%.
- Myocarditis or encephalitis are occasionally seen, and severe hypotension (dengue shock syndrome) might accompany DHF.

Differential diagnosis

- *See* 'Management of the febrile traveller', page 154.

Diagnosis

- The virus may occasionally be isolated from the blood, but rising antibody titres may be helpful.
- The white blood cell count is low, as is that of the platelets. In DHF the platelet count is very low (often $< 20 \times 10^9/l$), but disseminated intravascular coagulation is variable.

Treatment

- Treatment is symptomatic only, although DHF may require support with plasma, blood and platelet transfusions.

Prevention

- This is by eliminating the source of the mosquitoes, a strategy that has met with some success in certain areas.

Leishmaniasis

Causative agents

Visceral leishmaniasis (kala-azar)
- *Leishmania donovani* (various subspecies).

Cutaneous leishmaniasis

- *Leishmania major.*
- *Leishmania tropica.*
- *Leishmania aethiopica.*
- *Leishmania mexicana.*
- *Leishmania braziliensis* and others

Epidemiology and pathophysiology

- Kala-azar is widespread in the Mediterranean, Sudan, East Africa, India, China, South America and the Middle East.
- Cutaneous leishmaniasis is common throughout the tropics and subtropics.
- Sandflies of the genus *Phlebotomus* transmit the agents between infected carriers, including man, dog, fox and wild rodents.
- Visceral leishmaniasis has been diagnosed in AIDS patients and the symptoms are particularly severe in this setting.

Incubation period

- For kala-azar, 3–8 months, up to 10 years.
- For cutaneous leishmaniasis, 2–3 months, but up to 5 years.

Clinical features

Visceral leishmaniasis

- There can be a slow onset with low-grade fever, or a rapid onset of high fever. The fever rises rapidly and the ill patient usually develops hepatosplenomegaly with the spleen occasionally being massive. Anaemia is the rule and lymphadenopathy is common.
- Pigmentation of the face is a recognized but non-specific feature.
- A steady downhill course to death within weeks or months from a secondary infection, usually pneumonia, septicaemia or TB, is frequent.

Cutaneous leishmaniasis

- The lesions begin as single or multiple small papules, which grow up to 10 cm or more in diameter to form a rounded ulcer with raised edges and a granulomatous base.
- A seropurulent discharge may be present, and the lesion often has a hard central scab.
- The lesions are usually painless. Secondary infection can occur.
- If left untreated, the lesions persist for up to 1 year and heal to leave atrophic skin.

Differential diagnosis

- Visceral leishmaniasis is similar to a large range of acute and chronic infectious diseases, including malaria and typhoid as well as lymphoma.
- Cutaneous leishmaniasis must be distinguished from other skin ulcers.

Diagnosis

- Visceral leishmaniasis can be confirmed by direct demonstration or culture of the parasite from bone marrow or spleen (having confirmed normal clotting and platelets). Antibodies are also detected in serum. Pancytopenia, especially neutropenia, is almost invariable.
- In cutaneous leishmaniasis, the diagnosis should be confirmed by demonstrating the parasite in slit-skin smears by culture or staining. The smear is best taken through the ulcer edge.

Treatment

- Antimicrobial therapy for secondary infection, notably TB, pneumococcal infection and measles is required.
- Parenteral pentavalent antimony 20 mg per kg bodyweight up to 850 mg daily for 3 weeks is often effective in visceral leishmaniasis. Alternative drugs include pentamodine, allopurinal and paromomycin.
- Topical treatments have been tried for cutaneous leishmaniasis, such as curettage, heat and cryotherapy. Antimonials given intralesionally or parenterally are occasionally required. Topical paromomycin can also be effective.

Prevention

- Avoidance of sandfly bites.
- Insect repellants.

Rabies

Causative agent

- Rabies virus.

Epidemiology and pathophysiology

- There is a worldwide distribution, except in Australia, New Zealand, UK, Ireland, most of Scandinavia and Iceland. It is particularly common in the Indian subcontinent.
- There are two main pools of infection.

1 Rural (sylvatic) disease involves wild animals, such as foxes and bats; man is only rarely affected.
2 Urban disease is seen when cats and dogs are regularly involved; in this situation, man is at high risk, as for example in India.

- Human disease usually begins with a scratch or bite from an infected animal, or through transmission via mucous membranes. The virus cannot penetrate intact skin.
- Person-to-person spread is unlikely, although transmission by corneal graft has been reported.
- After the inoculation of virus, it spreads along the peripheral nerves to the CNS.
- Three reported cases in man in 18 countries in Europe in 1980 with 18 603 reported cases in animals in the same 18 countries in the same year.

Incubation period

- Usually 3–12 weeks, depending upon the site of the bite, although it can extend up to 19 years or be as short as 4 days.

Clinical features

- There may be tingling at the site of the wound initially, which may be accompanied by headache, sore throat and fever. After 2–10 days, the patient develops a state of anxiety, agitation, hyperactivity, difficulty in swallowing, leading to hydrophobia and hallucinations.
- Convulsive spasms are followed by paralysis, coma and death. The illness lasts 1–4 weeks depending on the intensive care given. There are three recorded survivors, all of whom received pre- or post-exposure prophylaxis.

Differential diagnosis

- This includes rabies hysteria, Guillain–Barré syndrome, poliomyelitis and encephalomyelitis.

Diagnosis

- Rabies antigen is demonstrable by immunoflourescent techniques from corneal smear, skin biopsies, and brain biopsies.
- Antibody is detectable in the serum during the illness.

Treatment

- Intensive care support is normally given but, when clinical symptoms develop, death is inevitable.

Prevention

- Immediate and thorough cleansing of bite/wound with soap and water and, if necessary, surgical toilet.
- Define the circumstances of the bite. Infection from an immunized animal is unlikely.
- Trace the animal's keeper if possible and have the animal quarantined. If it is still alive and well after 10 days, it is unlikely to be infected with rabies.
- Post-exposure active and passive immunization may be given if a bite or lick of a wound or mucous membrane occurred.

1 Active immunization: human diploid cell vaccine, 1 ml given im in 6 doses on days 0, 3, 7,14, 30 and 90, into the deltoid muscle.
2 Passive immunization: one dose of human rabies immunoglobulin, 20 iu/kg bodyweight, half of which is administered locally at the site of the wound and the other half is given im.

- Pre-exposure active immunization with human diploid cell vaccine should be offered to those workers exposed to animals which may have a greater risk of carrying rabies or those people travelling to remote areas in developing countries who may be at special risk, such as veterinary workers. Immunization involves 3 doses of 1 ml given at 0, 7 and 28 days.

Schistosomiasis (bilharzia)

Causative agents

- *Schistosoma haematobium*.
- *Schistosoma mansoni*.
- *Schistosoma japonicum*.
- Less commonly, other *Schistosoma* sp.

Epidemiology and pathophysiology

- *Schistosoma haematobium* is found in Egypt, Africa, Iran, Iraq, Syria, Yemen, South Arabia, Lebanon, Israel, Turkey, Cyprus and Portugal.
- *Schistosoma mansoni* is found in tropical Africa, the Nile Delta, Puerto Rico, Dominica and northern South America.
- *Schistosoma japonicum* is found in China, southern Japan and the Philippines, Thailand and Vietnam.
- Man is the only host of the fluke, which is transmitted from one infected person to another via the water snail (biomphalaria, bulimus, *Oncomelania* sp.). Person to person transmission is not possible.
- The water snail liberates cercariae into the water which penetrate the skin or mucus membranes of man and travel via the liver (to mature) to venules around the bladder or large bowel and grow into the adult worms. The adults produce eggs which are excreted into intestinal or bladder mucosa and thence into contaminated water. After the eggs hatch, the water snail is penetrated by the miracidia and thus the cycle is perpetuated.

incubation period

- 4–8 weeks.

Clinical features

- Tingling and itching (uncommonly) is noticed at the site of entry of the cercariae ('swimmer's itch').
- An acute illness consisting of headache, fever, aching muscles, abdominal pain, cough and, sometimes, pneumonia may follow. Hepatosplenomegaly and lymphadenopathy will be found ('Katayama fever'). Characteristically these symptoms subside after about a fortnight.
- Other symptoms are dependent upon the organism, but often include fatigue.
- Infection with *Schistosoma haematobium* is characterized by painless terminal haematuria. The haematuria is often made worse by exercise. In severe infections, frequency of micturition follows. Haemospermia, pyelonephritis and hydronephrosis may also complicate this infection, and there is a strong association with bladder cancer.
- Infection with *Schistosoma mansoni* is usually asymptomatic although a colitis with abdominal pain and frequent stools containing blood and mucus can be found. Hepatosplenomegaly occurs in prolonged and heavy infection, although jaundice is rare. Paraplegia from spinal lesions is a rare complication.

● Infection with *Schistosoma japonicum* is similar to that with *Schistosoma mansoni*.

Differential diagnosis

● As most cases are asymptomatic and detected only as incidental eosinophilia, the differential is large.
● *Schistosoma haemotobium* should be distinguished from urinary infection, stones and cancer.

Diagnosis

● There is a case for routine testing of those making prolonged visits to endemic areas.
● There is a non-specific antibody test that detects a schistosomal infection (including non-human schistosome contact).
● Microscopic examination of stool or, more sensitively, of rectal snips will identify the eggs of *Schistosoma mansoni* and *Schistosoma japonicum*. Microscopic examination of terminal urine for eggs of *Schistosoma haematobium* is sensitive when macroscopic or microscopic haematuria has been detected.
● Eosinophilia is found in most infections, especially in the acute syndrome in which high counts may be found.

Treatment

● Praziquantel 40 mg/kg orally as a single dose in infection with *Schistosoma haematobium*. For infection with *Schistosoma mansoni* and *Schistosoma japonicum*, 20 mg/kg, 12 hourly, for 3 days is required. Niridazole 25 mg/kg orally for 7 days in infections with *Schistosoma haematobium* is also effective.

Prevention

● Travellers should be warned to avoid all contact with fresh water.
● Hygienic disposal of faeces and urine in inhabitants of endemic areas is desirable.
● Attempts to kill the water snails have been made, not all of which have been successful.

Tetanus

Causative agent

- *Clostridium tetani.*

Epidemiology and pathophysiology

- It has a worldwide distribution.
- Spores of *Clostridium tetani* are found in soil contaminated by domestic animal faeces and can enter via the broken skin of contaminated wounds. Small but penetrating wounds are sufficient for penetration to occur and cases of ear infection have been documented.
- It may also occur in drug abusers who inject.
- The disease is seen in subjects of any age, although it is more common in older people.
- There were 9 cases and 2 deaths recorded in England and Wales in 1987. 8 cases were notified in 1990.

Incubation period

- 2–30 days, commonly 10.

Clinical features

- Initial symptoms of restlessness, irritability, stiffness or cramp may proceed to trismus (painful stiffening of the jaw muscles).
- Generalized rigidity progressively follows accompanied after 1–2 days by reflex spasms triggered by minor stimuli, such as noise.
- In severe cases, the rigidity is associated with tonic spasms causing arching of the back and the characteristic smiling expression (risus sardonicus). This may also cause pathological fractures, especially of the vertebrae.
- Death may occur from pneumonia, asphyxia or exhaustion.
- Involvement of the autonomic nervous system may also lead to profuse sweating, swinging fever, large fluctuations in blood pressure, tachycardia, and arrhythmias, which may further contribute to the death toll.
- The severity of illness is inversely proportional to the incubation period and therefore it influences mortality, which overall is about 5% with ideal therapy.
- Symptoms can persist for 2 months.

Differential diagnosis

● This includes dystonic drug reactions, especially those due to pheno-thiazines, tetany, dental abscess and rabies.

Diagnosis

● Diagnosis is usually made clinically.
● Isolation of the organism from a wound is difficult and not pathognomonic.

Treatment

● Initial surgical toilet of any wounds and the administration of parenteral benzylpenicillin or metronidazole is important.
● Human tetanus immunoglobulin 7–70 iu/kg is given im and a further intrathecal dose (up to 250 iu) may also help.
● Most patients require intensive care support; therapy is based on:

1 drugs such as diazepam for control of muscle spasms, and agents to control the autonomic dysfunction, e.g. propanalol or labetatol;
2 mechanical ventilation, together with the administration of muscle-paralysing agents, is frequently required.

● After recovery, tetanus vaccination is still necessary.

Prevention

● Primary immunization of infants and children is administered at the ages of 2, 3 and 4 months (*see* Chapter 17 on immunization).
● For adults and children over the age of 10 years, a primary course of immunization consists of the second dose being given 4–6 weeks after the first and the third dose 6 months after the second.
● Two reinforcing doses should be given at 10 year intervals. Immunity is then thought to be lifelong.
● For tetanus-prone wounds, management includes:

1 surgical toilet and antibiotics;
2 antitetanus immunoglobulin 250 iu (or 500 iu im if more than 24 hours have elapsed since injury), and the first of 3 vaccinations with tetanus toxoid if patients are not known to be fully immunized or if there is a greatly increased risk of contamination. The other two vaccinations should be given at monthly intervals thereafter;

3 probably no further tetanus toxoid in patients who have had a primary course or reinforcing dose of tetanus toxoid within 10 years, *unless* the wound is dirty in which case a single dose is sufficient;
4 a single reinforcing dose plus tetanus immunoglobulin if the wound is dirty in patients who have had a primary course or booster dose more than 10 years previously.

Yellow fever

Causative agent

● Yellow fever virus – a flavivirus (RNA).

Epidemiology and pathophysiology

● It is exclusively seen in tropical Africa and central and northern south America in rainforest areas.
● The arbovirus of yellow fever is spread to man by the bite of an infected mosquito of the genus *Aedes*.
● Lifelong immunity follows survival of the disease, and there is possibly some cross-immunity gained from previous infection with other flaviviruses.
● There is a sylvatic cycle in monkeys in which humans are occasionally victims having been bitten by a mosquito that previously fed on an infected monkey.
● An urban cycle may develop if infected subjects enter towns, and mosquitoes spread the disease from person to person.
● There have been no reported cases in England and Wales for the last 10 years.

Incubation period

● 3–6 days.

Clinical features

● The majority of infections are mild or symptomatic.
● In clinical disease there are 3 phases:

1 initial fever; followed by
2 a period of improvement; followed by
3 acute intoxication.

● The initial onset of fever may be accompanied by rigors, and the temperature is often highest on the first day.

- Headache, backache and bone pains may be followed by prostration, vomiting, epigastric pain, mental irritability and photophobia.
- The pulse rate falls more quickly than the temperature, and the disproportion between the pulse and temperature is often marked.
- At the end of 4 days, the temperature reaches normal as the second stage of the infection develops.
- In more serious cases, a third stage follows with the temperature rising, jaundice becoming pronounced, and bleeding may begin in various parts of the body.
- Meningo-encephalitis can occur.
- The overall mortality rate in such cases is 20–50%, although death rarely occurs in those who survive for 12 days or more.

Differential diagnosis

- The initial feverish illness has a wide differential.
- Fever *and* jaundice in combination are uncommon in other conditions except for glandular fever, leptospirosis, typhoid, malaria, cholangitis and other viral haemorrhagic fevers.

Diagnosis

- The virus or rising antibody titres may be detected in blood samples.
- The patient may also have leucopenia and clotting abnormalities, and have abnormalitites on liver and renal function tests.

Treatment

- Treatment is supportive only.

Prevention

- Vaccination given at recognized centres confers immunity for at least 10 years. It is a live attenuated vaccine and highly effective following a single dose.

The notifiable viral haemorrhagic fevers (VHF)

Causative agents

- Lassa fever virus – an arenavirus (RNA).
- Congo–Crimea virus – a nairovirus (RNA).
- Ebola and Marburg viruses – filoviruses (RNA).

Epidemiology

- Lassa virus is endemic in the multimammate rat (*Mastomys natalensis*) in rural subsaharan West and Central Africa. Transmission to man occurs through direct contamination by fomites, especially from rat urine. Person-to-person spread is usually through body fluids, although transmission via the respiratory route is possible.
- Congo–Crimea virus is endemic throughout the tropics and subtropics of the Old World as far east as India. It infects wild and domestic animals and spreads to man mainly through the bite of ticks.
- Marburg virus has been recognized only rarely since the first outbreak in Germany associated with imported green (Vervet) monkeys. Little is known of the epidemiology other than it is present in South and East Africa.
- Ebola virus infection is also found in East Africa, in Sudan and Zaire, but nothing is known of its epidemiology other than large outbreaks are observed centred on hospitals. Person-to-person transmission, therefore, is most likely through body fluids.

Incubation period

- Lassa fever virus: 6–21 days.
- Congo–Crimea virus: 3–6   days.
- Ebola virus: 2–21 days.
- Marburg virus: 3–9   days.

Clinical features

- These four infections have the characteristics of a high mortality rate, possible person-to-person spread and, frequently, a non-specific onset.
- Lassa fever is frequently asymptomatic, but in those with clinically apparent disease, chest, back and abdominal pain, sore throat, cough, vomiting and diarrhoea, and conjunctivitis may variably by present. Facial oedema is an uncommon but relatively specific feature. Progression to multisystem failure, generalized oedema and bleeding is seen in the second week when death can occur. The mortality rate of untreated symptomatic disease is 15–25%.
- Congo–Crimea haemorrhagic fever is frequently asymptomatic. When severe symptomatic disease occurs, disseminated intravascular coagulation and hepatitis dominate the picture; there is a 20–50% mortality rate.

- Marburg and Ebola virus infections are similar, presenting with a 'flu-like illness. Vomiting and diarrhoea appear over the next 2–3 days, followed by a generalized maculopapular rash. Disseminated intravascular coagulation is seen in the severe cases in which death occurs early in the second week of illness. Mortality rates of 30% for Marburg disease and 70% in Ebola infection have been observed.

Differential diagnosis

- *See* 'Management of the febrile traveller', page 104.

Diagnosis

- It is the duty of every doctor seeing a patient with a fever who has returned from an area where VHF is endemic to discuss the possible diagnosis with the local CCDC, one of the designated isolation units for VHF, or the Communicable Disease Surveillance Centre at Colindale (081 200 6868) or the Communicable Disease Centre, Scotland (041 946 7120).
- Suspicion for Lassa fever should be high if the patient is febrile and, within 3 weeks of onset, visited rural West or Central Africa, particularly the savannah or Sahel regions. However, as malaria is such a common cause of fever in this circumstance, this diagnosis should be excluded if the patient has presented to a hospital. A film should be made from blood taken using a gown, mask, visor and gloves, the patient being isolated immediately. The film should be dealt with using strict precautions. If malaria is confirmed, the patient should be isolated in a normal infectious disease unit until the fever has disappeared. If the film is negative, the doctor should discuss with the above authorities the need for transportation to a specialized unit.
- As Congo–Crimea, Ebola and Marburg haemorrhagic fevers are far less common, and much less predictable in their geography; their diagnosis is normally considered when further features of an unknown VHF are present, such as abnormal clotting tests.
- The diagnosis of Lassa, Congo–Crimea, Ebola or Marburg haemorrhagic fever is established in a high security unit, using tissue culture of body fluids and antibody tests.
- Suspicion of a VHF should be raised if the patient presents with a febrile influenza-like illness with conjunctivitis and bleeding into skin mucous membranes and/or internal organs.

Treatment

- Suspected cases should be isolated in the units designated by the Department of Health (DoH).

- Lassa fever will respond to therapy with ribavirine given orally or parenterally. The other three conditions can be managed only symptomatically.

Prevention

- Little can be done for the person who has to visit a rural area endemic for these conditions other than to maintain as strict a regimen of hygiene as possible.

Common intestinal parasites

Causative agents

Hookworm
- *Necator americanus.*
- *Ancylostoma duodenale.*

Roundworm
- *Ascaris lumbricoides.*
- *Strongyloidicesis.*
- *Strongyloides stercoralis.*

Whipworm
- *Trichuris trichiuria.*

Tapeworms
- *Taenia* sp.

Epidemiology

- These infections are diseases of poor hygiene and infrequently found in Western visitors to the tropics, although some indigenous people returning to remote villages may be affected. These infections extend throughout the tropics and subtropics.
- Hookworm and *Strongyloides* infect humans by penetration of the skin after the larvae hatch in moist soil.
- The *Ascaris*, *Trichuris* and *Taenia* spp. cause infection after the ingestion of contaminated food or water.
- Millions of inhabitants of the tropics, especially children, are infected.
- *Strongyloides* may persist for 40 years or more, for example, as seen in prisoners of war held in the Far East during the Second World War.

Incubation period

- Hookworm: 4–6 weeks.
- Roundworm: 2 months.
- *Strongyloides:*   4 weeks.
- Whipworm: 1–3 months.
- Tapeworm: 2 months.

Clinical features

- Most light infections are asymptomatic.
- Migrations of hookworm larvae may cause dyspnoea, cough, wheeze and fever (Löffler's syndrome). Heavy gut infection may lead to anaemia.
- Löffler's syndrome may also be caused by roundworm. Heavy intestinal infection can lead to weight loss, and intestinal and bilary obstruction.
- Infection with *Strongyloides* may initially cause abdominal pains, severe watery diarrhoea, weight loss and an urticarial rash. As the larvae are able to penetrate the gut wall, recurrent tissue invasion occurs from worms releasing eggs within the gut which hatch before being passed in the faeces. These organisms cause a recurrent round or linear urticarial rash on the lower trunk and thigh ('larva currens'). The gut stage is normally asymptomatic. If an infected patient is *immunosuppressed* with steroids or diabetes, for instance, the hyper-infection syndrome may ensue with diarrhoea, hypotension, pneumonitis, meningitis, Gram-negative septicaemia and death.
- Whipworm is rarely symptomatic, although very heavy infections may cause poor weight gain and diarrhoea in children.
- Tapeworm infection confined to the gut is usually asymptomatic apart from minor digestive problems, although live proglottids may be passed through the anus periodically. Infection is acquired through eating beef or pork contaminated with immature stages of the parasite (scolices). If the eggs of the pork tapeworm (*Taenia solium*) are accidentally eaten, cysticercosis develops with tissue invasion leading to the deposition of the cysts within many tissues, including the brain. Epilepsy may develop, as well as hydrocephalus and focal neurological signs.

Diagnosis

- All infections can be diagnosed by examination of fresh stool for eggs or larvae. *Strongyloides* identification can be difficult and may require stool culture, or isolation of larvae from duodenal/jejunal juice obtained by swallowing absorbent string in a gelatin capsule ('string test'). There is also an antibody test.

- Cysticercosis can be confimed by antibody testing, and typical changes are seen on CT scanning.
- In tissue invasion phases there is often a raised eosinophil count which can be very high. Patchy chest X-ray changes characterize Löfflers syndrome.

Treatment

- Mebendazole for hookworm, roundworm or whipworm, 200 mg, 12 hourly, for 3 days irrespective of weight. Not suitable for young children.
- *Strongyloides* will respond to thiabendazole 25 mg/kg, 12 hourly, for 2 days although side effects are significant. Treatment may have to be extended for 2 weeks in the hyper-infection syndrome. Labendazole is an alternative.
- Tapeworm responds to a single dose of praziquantel 20 mg/kg. Niclosomide, 2 g for adults, 1 g for children 2–6 years old, and 500 mg for children under 2 years, is also effective as a single dose but it is best given with an anti-emetic to prevent cysticercosis.
- The scolices of cysticercosis can be killed by praziquantel 50 mg/kg divided into 3 doses daily for 14 days, although steroids also have a place to prevent further seizures as the organism dies.

Prevention

- Good food and water hygiene (*see* section on diarrhoea, page 52) and the strict use of shoes out of doors will prevent infection. All meat must be thoroughly cooked to kill tapeworm.
- Ex prisoners of war held captive in the Far East are routinely screened for *Strongyloides* at centres designated by the DoH.
- Patients from the tropics and subtropics should be screened for *Strongyloides* if steroids or other immunosuppressives are to be given.

CHAPTER 15

Pyrexia of unknown origin, glandular fever and other infections causing lymphadenopathy

THE diagnoses of febrile illnesses are only rarely difficult within the setting of a district general hospital. After having taken a thorough history and examined the patient carefully, a short working differential diagnosis is usually possible. Even if that is not possible, appropriate investigation will lead to the diagnosis in most cases. A significant number of diagnoses of pyrexia of unknown origin (PUO) arise from inappropriate initial management. In this chapter, several diseases with the characteristics of associated lymphadenopathy are also described.

Pyrexia of unknown orgin

Common causative agents

Viruses
- CMV.
- EBV.
- HIV.

Bacteria
- *Mycobacterium tuberculosis.*
- *Brucella* sp.
- *Mycoplasma pneumoniae.*
- *Salmonella typhi.*
- *Coxiella burnetii.*
- The agents of infective endocarditis.

Protozoa
- *Toxoplasma gondii.*
- Malaria.

Others
- Drugs.
- Malignancies.

- Autoimmune disease.
- Vasculitis.
- Factitious fever.
- Deep pus.

Epidemiology and pathophysiology

- PUO is defined as the presence of fever >37.5°C, for at least 2 weeks, the cause of which remains unclear after at least 1 week's hospital investigation.
- This definition excludes the majority of minor self-limiting viral infections which are so common in the community.
- The most likely cause is influenced by the age, sex and race of the patient; TB is the most likely cause in an Asian patient, whilst EBV infection is common in teenage Caucasians.

Clinical features

- CMV infection frequently presents with no more than fever and lymphadenopathy in the immunocompetent, although more extensive disease is seen in the immunocompromised. Viral culture and antigen testing of urine is diagnostic.
- A similar onset may be seen in young and middle-aged adults with EBV infection. Approximately 10% will be monospot-negative and specific virological testing may be required.
- Brucellosis is often quoted as a disease in this context, but it is quite rare in the UK. Acute infection causes fever, headache, arthralgia, lymphadenopathy and hepatosplenomegaly to some degree. The organism can be cultured from the blood in this situation. When chronic infection supervenes, the illness can be very non-specific, inducing fevers, sweats and weight loss. Antibody testing can confirm this diagnosis, which is also suggested by the presence of granulomas in the liver. The majority of cases are imported.
- Mycoplasma and coxiella (Q fever) infections can be difficult to diagnose. Although both may cause pneumonia and pneumonitis, non-specific presentations can be found including a glandular fever-like illness, granulomatous hepatitis, myocarditis, and, in the case of *Coxiella*, endocarditis.
- *Toxoplasma gondii* infection does not always produce lymphadenopathy and splenomegaly. Whilst the young and middle-aged are most commonly affected, no age is exempt. Toxoplasma antibody testing should always be considered to exclude this very common infection.

- As long as a travel history has been taken, malaria and typhoid will not be missed. Typhoid can present a month or more after return, and several UK-acquired cases are notified each year. Malaria may cause illness many years after the last visit to an endemic area.
- All fevers are not due to infection; common examples of those that are not include those induced by lymphoma, retroperitoneal sarcoma, systemic lupus erythematosus, giant cell arteritis, and drugs, such as phenytoin. Patients may also simulate a fever (Munchhausen's syndrome).
- These and other similar conditions should be considered according to the circumstance and diagnosed appropriately.
- CT and ultrasound imaging may be useful whereas radionuclide (e.g. gallium) scanning is less likely to help.

Differential diagnosis

- Few feverish illnesses will fall within the strict definition of PUO if the initial history, examination and investigation are carried out with attention to detail. Obvious examples from history include the identification of a patient at risk for HIV infection or recognition of the fact that recent surgery may have lead to an abdominal abscess or thrombo-embolic disease.
- Initial investigation does not always have to be extensive if careful thought is given to the clues derived from the history and examination. In the majority of febrile patients in whom the diagnosis is not immediately obvious, chest X-ray, full blood count, LFT, ESR, 3 blood cultures, urine culture and a monospot test will normally lead to the identification of the infection. In particular, pneumonia and TB may present with very subtle signs, as may a UTI. If the white cell count is raised with a neutrophilia, a bacterial infection should be sought, whereas a normal or low white count suggests a viral aetiology. Important exceptions are typhoid and brucellosis.

Diagnosis

- Examination of the patient should be thorough and may be repeated many times if a subtle progression of signs is to be detected. All of the clothing may have to be removed if a small patch of erysipelas is to be recognized. A subtle murmur may be apparent only after numerous careful auscultations of the heart sounds, thus revealing infective endocarditis or atrial myxoma.

- Many facets of HIV infection can be associated with non-specific febrile illness. The diagnosis depends on an initial suspicion. Seroconversion illness will then be readily confirmed by the detection of viral antigen in the blood. Once HIV antibody test is known to be positive, the diseases mentioned previously (*see* HIV infection, page 140) may be pursued.
- TB appears at the top of most lists as the diagnosis that most commonly eludes detection. The elderly, immigrants, alcoholics, diabetics and the immunocompromised are all particularly prone to this infection, which should be sought with vigour. In the context of PUO, extrapulmonary disease and, particularly, TB lymphadenitis, miliary TB and TB meningitis can be difficult to diagnose. Lymphadenitis affects young and middle-aged adult immigrants particularly, in whom minor cervical or hilar lymphadenopathy may be the only sign. Lymph-node biopsy will establish the diagnosis. Meningitis is often extremely subtle in its presentation, headaches or fever being the only features of early disease. Meningism and neurological signs appear relatively late. The diagnosis of miliary TB may be even more difficult. Sputum, gastric washings and early morning urine microscopy and cultures may identify the organism, and chest X-ray changes are sometimes suggestive. Liver biopsy is probably the most useful test, especially if there are minor abnormalities in the LFT, such as an aspartate aminotransferase level a few units above the normal range. Granulomas and even acid-fast bacilli, in a proportion, will be seen. Mantoux testing and the ESR may suggest the diagnosis but can be unreactive in extensive disease. Cryptic miliary TB in the elderly may be particularly subtle in presentation and a trial of specific antituberculous drugs (isoniazid, pyrazinamide, and ethambutol) may eventually be required.

Treatment

- The first rule in the treatment of PUO is *do not* prescribe drugs speculatively unless the patient's illness is severe and deterioration is likely. Fever, however severe and prolonged, is not in itself a sufficient reason to warrant antibiotic therapy in the absence of a diagnosis. All conditions mentioned have their specific therapy (as indicated elsewhere in this book). On rare occasions, a diagnosis may not have been reached after extensive investigation. In some cases, the patient remains well and therapy may be withheld until the diagnosis is reached or the fever finally disappears. If a steady deterioration is observed, antituberculous therapy is often given on the basis that this has been shown to be the most common cause of this condition. Steroids may also be considered since autoimmune and vasculitic disease may also be associated with this type of presentation.

Glandular fever (infectious mononucleosis)

Causative agents

- EBV.
- CMV.
- HIV.
- *Toxoplasma gondii.*

Epidemiology and pathophysiology

- EBV-related disease is most commonly seen in teenagers and young adults although no age-group is exempt, and transmission between children at nurseries is frequent. The virus is transmitted by close contact, including kissing and sexual intercourse, and possibly by droplet. More infection is seen in the autumn and winter. Clinically apparent infection is estimated to be approximately 200 per 100 000 population per year.
- CMV is much less common as a cause of disease than EBV in the immunocompetent. Transmission has been recognized by a variety of routes including transplacentally, by contamination with vaginal secretions at birth, blood transfusions, sexual intercourse and possibly fomites. This organism causes major disease in the immuno-compromised and also is the cause of congenital abnormalities in approximately 6 per 10 000 livebirths.
- HIV is considered in Chapter 13 (page 140).
- *Toxoplasma gondii* also causes disease, most commonly in young adults. It is particularly common in rural areas. Infection is acquired either from the ingestion of oocysts passed in infected cat faeces and contaminating the environment, such as sandpits or salad vegetables, or from eating poorly cooked ('rare') meat, as is common practice in France (France has a particularly high rate of infection). By adulthood, there is evidence of past infection in 30% of the population. The life-cycle of the parasite is poorly understood, but involves sexual reproduction in the gut of cats, ingestion of oocysts by other animals and re-infection of cats when the meat of infected animals is eaten. Congenital infection is relatively common although there is some evidence that fetal malformations are less frequent than was previously thought.

Clinical features

- Glandular fever refers to a febrile illness in which lymphadenopathy is found. Infectious mononucleosis a term that is often used inter-changeably with glandular fever and refers to the common finding of a large number of atypical mononuclear cells (which are actually activated T lymphocytes) in the bloiod of patients with some of these conditions. The clinical manifestations of EBV infection have already been described in the section on tonsillitis (Chapter 3, page 13).

- CMV is rarely a cause of tonsillitis and in most clinically manifest infections in the immunocompetent it is associated with a prolonged febrile illness with generalized lymphadenopathy. If infection occurs in pregnancy, 50% of infants will be infected, of whom 1 in 4 show symptoms. These may include microcephaly, blindness, motor problems and mental retardation. Deafness can occur many years after birth and may be the sole feature. An acute multisystem involvement may be found at birth, which may include hepatitis, respiratory distress, a petechial rash, convulsions and hepatosplenomegaly. The mortality is high. If infection occurs at birth, the only consequence will be prolonged urinary excretion without symptoms.
- HIV infection is described in Chapter 13.
- Acute toxoplasmosis has a reputation of being a prolonged illness, although the majority (90%) of infections are asymptomatic. The most frequent manifestation is cervical lymphadenopathy without fever. Generalized lymphadenopathy, fever, rash, pharyngitis and hepatosplenomegaly are found in only a minority of infections. Extremely rare infections presenting with multisystem disease have been described. Symptoms last 1–2 months in the majority, but can occasionally extend beyond 1 year. Chorioretinitis can occur after acute infection, with some visual impairment. Unilateral eye involvment is the rule with yellow or white cottonwool patches seen on the retina. Congenital infection may result from infection during pregnancy, and is most severe in the first trimester with abortion, stillbirth and fetal malformations in some. Only 25–65% of infected women will transmit the infection to the infant, and 10–30% of these infants will have disease. Most manifestations are clinically mild, but can include chorioretinitis and other causes of blindness, mental retardation, epilepsy, microcephaly, hydrocephalus, cerebral calcification and a multisystem disease similar to that described for congenital CMV infection.

Differential diagnosis

- A wide range of infections can occasionally cause a glandular fever-like illness and include *Mycoplasma pneumoniae, Coxiella burnetii,* tuberculous lymphadenitis, cat-scratch fever, lymphoma and lymphoblastic leukaemia.

Diagnosis

- EBV infection can be detected by the heterophile antibody test (e.g. Paul–Bunnell or monospot) looking for antibodies that agglutinate sheep or horse red cells. This is positive in 90% of adult infections and 50% of those in childhood, although the test may only become reactive after 2 weeks. Specific antibodies directed against the early antigen (EA), VCA and EBNA can be used to identify the rest. Typically anti-EA and anti-VCA appear in acute infection, with anti-EBNA appearing during recovery. Acute infection is normally confirmed with an IgM anti-VCA.

- CMV infection is confirmed by detection of virus or viral antigen (by the detection of early antigen by fluorescent foci [DEAFF] test) by culture of body fluids, especially urine. This can also be applied to the infant. Antibody testing is unreliable save as an indication of past infection. In HIV seroconversion illness the p24 antigen test confirms the diagnosis.

- The serological diagnosis of toxoplasmosis is fraught with difficulties. High antibody titres may persist for many years whereas acute infection may be associated with very low titres. Most laboratories use one of several IgG antibody tests as a screening method (immunofluorescent antibody test and latex agglutinating antibody) and a test for IgM antibody (immunofluorescent, sandwich and immunosorbent assay) in those with high IgG titres. The dye test is very specific and used for confirmation. Serum antibody tests are unhelpful in ocular disease, although they can be found in the aqueous humour. The IgM test is used routinely to detect affected pregnancies in countries with a high prevalance (e.g. France), and IgM antibodies in neonatal blood will confirm congenital infection. Amniocentesis, fetal blood sampling and ultrasound scanning are helpful for planning therapy in affected pregnancies.

- The most common non-specific abnormality found in these infections is a high number of atypical mononuclear cells, which in EBV infection may amount to 30% or more of the total white cell count. In any case, there is often a high lymphocyte count in this infection. These findings are less frequent in the other infections described, in which a normal or low white cell count may be found. Additional haematological abnormalities in EBV infection may include cold-agglutinin-mediated haemolytic anaemia.

- LFT abnormalities are particularly common in EBV infection, where a concomitant rise in alkaline phosphatase and aminotransferase levels is seen. CMV may also do this.

Treatment

- Only acute toxoplasmosis is amenable to antibiotic therapy, although this is uncommonly used because of the poor rate of response and the relatively toxic nature of these drugs. Fansidar 2 tablets daily in adult, or spiramycin 1 g, 12 hourly, have both been used for up to 4 weeks. They are normally only given in severe or prolonged infection and for eye disease.
- The management of toxoplasmosis in pregnancy is especially problematic given the difficulty in predicting the pregnancies likely to be most severely affected. In France, spiramycin 3 g daily in 3–4 divided doses seems to reduce the damage caused by this infection. Fansidar has been tried after the first trimester. Some pregnancies have been aborted, although this is very controversial.
- Although there is no specific antimicrobial therapy that will affect the progress of EBV infection, steroids occasionally have a role (e.g. 0.6 mg/kg prednisolone daily) in complicated disease, such as upper airways obstruction, haemolytic anaemia and aggressive acute infection.
- CMV in the immunocompetent is exceedingly rare as a cause of severe disease, and the known effective agents, ganciclovir and foscarnet are reserved for disease in the immunocompromised.
- As CMV infection in pregnancy is rarely detected, abortion is not commonly an option.
- HIV glandular fever illness is not amenable to specific therapy.

Prevention

- HIV has been discussed previously (page 140).
- There is little prospect of preventing the spread of EBV and CMV at present.
- Toxoplasmosis is avoidable by preventing the fouling of sandpits and vegetables by cats, the thorough washing of salad vegetables and the prolonged cooking of meat.

Listeriosis

Causative agent

- *Listeria monocytogenes*, a Gram-positive bacillus.

Epidemiology and pathophysiology

- The organism is widely distributed in soil.

- Contaminated foods, especially soft cheese, unpasteurized dairy products, chicken and pre-packed salads are the main source of infection. After ingestion, a period of asymptomatic bowel colonization may occur.
- The organism can grow at refrigeration temperatures (4°C).
- Infection is mainly seen in the very young, very old, pregnancy and the immunocompromised, although the immunocompetent can also be infected.
- The peak period of infection is the autumn.
- 250–300 cases are reported in England and Wales each year, of which approximately one-third are related to pregnancy.

Incubation period

- 7–30 days.

Clinical features

- Several syndromes are recognized.
- Focal infections may be recognized in many organs, including eyes, pharynx, salivary glands, bones, joints and endocarditis.
- Meningo-encephalitis can present as an acute meningitis or encephalitis at any age.
- Infection in pregnancy can be very mild with symptoms suggestive of UTI. Miscarriage and premature labour can occur.
- Neonatal infection may be the result of infection in pregnancy. Neonatal death or a severe septicaemic illness at or soon after birth can result. Meningitis occurs at about 1 week of age.
- A non-specific febrile illness can be seen in the immunocompromised.

Differential diagnosis

- The meningitis and encephalitis presentations are similar to infections caused by the more common bacteria and viruses.
- Neonatal infection is similar to that due to group B streptococci or E. coli.

Diagnosis

- Diagnosis relies firstly on suspicion in those belonging to groups known to be at risk.
- The organism is readily grown from various body fluids, including blood and CSF. Growth can be slow.
- In CNS syndromes, the CSF may contain a mixture of lymphocytes and neutrophils, with a low glucose and high protein.

Treatment

- A variety of antibiotics including ampicillin, erythromycin and tetracycline can be effective. Ampicillin and gentamicin may act synergistically. Chloramphenicol may be effective in meningitis. At least two weeks' therapy is required.

Prevention

- Food hygiene is the key to prevention. Refrigerator temperatures must be kept below 4°C.
- Pregnant women in particular should avoid contact with infected animals, soft cheeses and paté.

Brucellosis

Causative agents

- *Brucella abortus*.
- *Brucella melitensis*.
- *Brucella suis*.
  (Gram-negative bacilli)

Epidemiology and pathophysiology

- There is a world-wide distribution of these organism. Although the Mediterranean basin and South America have a particularly high incidence of infection.
- Various species are found in cattle (*Brucella abortus*), goats (*Brucella melitensis*) and pigs (*Brucella suis*). They also occur in dogs, oxen and camels.
- It is rare in the UK, due to vaccination of calves and the slaughter of infected cattle.
- The infection is commonest in veterinary surgeons, abattoir workers and farmers who inhale or ingest contaminated material and are in direct contact with infected animals.
- It is also transmitted in unpasteurized milk or milk products.
- 18 cases were identified in England and Wales in 1987.
- In Europe, brucellosis is a typical Mediterranean disease of the rural population, especially those involved with animals. It also affects the tourist population, particularly those consuming fresh cheese and unpasteurized milk. It is particularly prevalent in France (about 500 cases per year), Greece (about 1750 cases a year), Italy (about 3000 cases a year) and Spain (7400 cases in 1981).

Incubation period

● 1–8 weeks.

Clinical features

● The onset may be sudden (33%) or gradual (67%) with fever sometimes lasting several months. Night sweats are common as the fever relapses and remits. Other symptoms include sore throat, cough, headache, arthralgia, insomnia, depression and abdominal pain.
● An erythematous rash, weight loss, lymphadenopathy and hepatosplenomegaly may be detected on examination.
● Complications include arthritis, spondylitis, neuritis, meningo-encephalitis, depression, endocarditis, hepatitis and orchitis. Virtually any organ can be affected.

Diagnosis

● This depends on which of the many possible sites is involved.
● Blood cultures taken during a febrile episode will have 70% yield, increased to 90% by marrow culture. The samples should not be discarded for at least 6 weeks.
● Antibodies are detectable from the 2nd week of infection. Owing to low sensitivity and low specificity, a battery of tests is usually carried out.
● The white blood cell count sometimes reveals neutropenia and lymphocytosis.
● Granulomata will be found on liver biopsy.

Treatment

● Two therapeutic agents are normally required.
● Tetracycline 7 mg/kg, 6 hourly, for 6 weeks with streptomycin 13 mg/kg daily for 3 weeks is a well-tried and effective regimen.
● Doxycycline 3 mg/kg and rifampicin 10 mg/kg daily for 6 weeks is probably more effective.

Prevention

● Vaccination of calves and slaughter of infected cattle, with the pasteurization of milk has proven successful in the UK.
● A similar procedure can also be applied to pigs and goats.

Cat-scratch fever

Causative agent

- An, as yet, uncharacterized bacillus.

Epidemiology and pathophysiology

- The bite, scratch or lick from a cat, or other animal, which itself shows no sign of disease is the usual cause.
- The disease mainly affects children and young adults and is most common in the colder months.

Incubation period

- 14 days approximately.

Clinical features

- After the scratch, a papule or pustule forms on the skin 3–10 days later.
- Headache, fever and, sometimes, a rash develops in 30%.
- Regional lymphadenopathy is the major manifestation lasting 2–4 months. The multiple lymph nodes can involve many sites. Suppuration of the node can occur in 10% of cases.
- Rarely, encephalitis, myelitis or inflammation of the spinal nerves, and a chronic rash similar to Kaposi's sarcoma have been seen.

Differential diagnosis

- Any cause of lymphadenopathy.

Diagnosis

- Biopsy of affected lymph nodes reveals typical histology and the organism may be seen with silver stain.
- A specific skin sensitivity test is available, but it is not recommended because of the risk of transmission of other diseases.

Treatment

- There is no specific treatment.

Prevention

- Thorough cleansing of animal-inflicted wounds may halt infection.

CHAPTER 16

Miscellaneous diseases recently defined as having an infective aetiology

ALTHOUGH the manifestations of the diseases described in this chapter have ben recognized for many years, their infectious aetiology has, at least for haemolytic uraemic syndrome (HUS) and Lyme disease, been delineated only within the last decade or so. The causes of myalgic encephalomyelitis and Kawasaki disease have yet to be elucidated, but eventually they will be linked more firmly to infectious agents. The conditions described here are only a few of those being investigated in infectious disease research, serving to emphasize the diversity of symptoms that microorganisms can cause. It is possible that a large proportion of today's 'idiopathic' conditions, such as inflammatory bowel disease, autoimmune diseases and even atheromatous arteries, may have an infectious basis.

Myalgic encephalomyelitis

Causative agents

● Unknown, but thought to be EBV or enteroviruses (especially Coxsackie B virus).

Epidemiology and pathophysiology

● Also known as chronic fatigue syndrome, post-viral fatigue syndrome, Royal Free Disease, Akureyri disease, Iceland disease, and Otago mystery disease. This condition has been recognized in one form or other for at least 70 years.
● It is thought to be extremely common, although the exact incidence is unknown.
● Peak incidence is at age 30–40 years, although no age-group is spared.
● There seems to be no ethnic differences.
● A higher incidence is found in women, health workers, teachers, athletes, dancers, hairdressers and people employed in occupations involving strenuous exercise or prolonged periods of standing.

- Parents of young children are also prone.
- Secondary cases in the same family have been reported in 25% of cases.

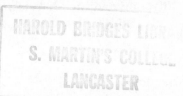

Incubation period

- 2–7 days in the acute form.

Clinical features

- Typically, the patient has been perfectly fit and well until they experience an acute 'flu-like illness, but, instead of recovery, they begin to experience the following symptoms.
- Muscle fatigability is characteristic, and extreme tiredness after varying degrees of physical effort. The muscle groups affected may not only be weak, but also tender to touch.
- Fasciculation, myoclonic jerks, and tender nodules in the muscles may occasionally be found on examination.
- Autonomic disturbances can give rise to poor vasomotor control, characterized by orthostatic tachycardias, low blood pressure, extreme sensitivity to heat and cold, drenching sweats and hypoglycaemic attacks.
- The nervous system is affected in a variety of ways, including emotional lability, headaches, depression, loss of concentration, difficulty in focusing, poor memory, and panic attacks.
- Sensory symptoms may include paraesthesia.
- The lymphatic system may be involved leading to recurrent lymphadenopathy, usually cervical, but sometimes it is generalized.
- Gastrointestinal disturbances may lead to symptoms similar to irritable bowel syndrome, including diarrhoea and/or constipation, bloating and abdominal discomfort.
- The ears may be affected giving rise particularly to tinnitus, deafness or increased sensitivity to noise.
- Various other associations include thyroiditis, parotitis, orchitis, arthritis, recurrent bacterial conjunctivitis, skin rashes, and disturbances of micturition have been reported.
- The symptoms and signs may vary in intensity from episode to episode. Relapses and remissions may recur over a number of years.
- Recovery does occur, but may take several years and a few remain chronically ill.
- Relapses may occur in relation to hormonal changes, changes in the weather, undue physical or mental strain, or *post* surgery or after injections, and drugs.

Differential diagnosis

● All other chronic debilitating illnesses should be excluded, such as hypothyroidism, diabetes, malignancies, endogenous depression, myopathies, myasthenia gravis, toxoplasmosis and brucellosis.

Diagnosis

● The diagnosis is difficult to establish because the symptoms are so diverse and, often, non-specific.
● The following investigations may be helpful, but they are not diagnostic.

1 Full blood count is usually normal.
2 The biochemical profile is usually normal.
3 Microbiological tests are worthwhile in order to exclude other infections as appropriate, such as rubella, CMV, EBV and *Toxoplasma*.

● A characteristic pattern of anti-VCA positivity and anti-EBNA negativity may be found on testing for EBV.
● Coxsackie B virus IgM is positive in 20% of patients.

Treatment

● Rest is advisable during acute illness or in relapses.
● Drugs are best avoided, as is alcohol, although antidepressants may help those with a subsequent reactive depression.
● Graded exercise may be started after the acute phase, the amount of activity should be designed to fall short of that which produces fatigue.
● Meditation and other non-specific aids to well-being can be tried.
● More contentious and unproven therapies include anticandidal treatment and diets, dietary supplements, extraction of teeth fillings, colonic lavage and prolonged sedation.
● A self-help group has been set up to support sufferers: The Myalgic Encephalomyelitis Association, P.O. Box 8, Standford-le-Hope, Essex, SS17 8EX.

Prevention

● This is not possible because the aetiology is not known.

Lyme disease

Causative agent

- *Borrelia burgdorferi*, a spirochaete.

Epidemiology and pathophysiology

- The organism is widespread in temperate and Mediterranean-type climates worldwide, including continental Europe, Australia, China, the USA (especially New England and California) and the UK.
- Cases in the UK are particularly associated with visits to the New Forest (Hampshire) and the lowlands of Scotland, although conditions suitable for transmission of the disease exist in many other areas.
- The infection is endemic in deer, sheep, cattle and, possibly, small mammals, rodents and birds. The organism is transmitted to man by the bite of an ixodeid tick, which transfers to its host from tall grass and low scrub, attaching mainly to the legs.
- Risk groups include farm and forestry workers, joggers and orienteering enthusiasts. The peak months of infection occur in the spring and summer.

Incubation period

- 3–30 days.

Clinical features

- The clinical features can loosely be divided into 3 stages, as follows.

1 Stage I occurs in approximately 50% of patients and presents as a central papule or macule from which spreads an erythematous ring – erythema chronicum migrans (ECM). This lesion can be very large (up to 70 cm in diameter) and last for many months. Multiple, smaller secondary rings may also develop subsequently. Associated systemic features can include fever, myalgia, lymphadenopathy and malaise, or occasionally a severe illness with CNS, lymphatic and hepatic features, which often fluctuates in severity.

2 Stage II disease often presents without a previous stage I illness and appears weeks or months after initial infection. The symptoms may overlap with ECM. Manifestations can include a flitting poly-arthralgia, aseptic meningitis, encephalitis, cranial nerve palsy (especially VII), myelitis, radiculitis and peripheral neuropathy.

Transient cardiac conduction defects are also well recognized. Although most of these problems will resolve spontaneously after several weeks or months, fatalities from severe CNS and cardiac involvement have been reported.

3 Months or years into the infection, stage III disease will become apparent; it is not necessarily preceded by stages I and II. The best recognized manifestation is a symmetrical large joint polyarthritis which can be found in up to 50% of untreated patients. This can be severe and recur for up to 8 years. Chronic neurologic sequelae, including encephalitis, dementia, myelitis and myocarditis, have also been described.

Differential diagnosis

- This can be wide.
- The rash of ECM may be confused with other rashes.
- The aseptic meningitis is often confused with viral meningitis.
- The facial palsy is often confused with idiopathic Bell's palsy.
- Arthritis may be ascribed to one of the other causes of 'seronegative' or 'reactive' arthropathy.
- Congenital infection leading to multisystem disease is recognized.

Diagnosis

- Diagnosis depends initially on clinical suspicion because it is still an uncommonly detected condition.
- The organism can occasionally be grown or demonstrated histologically from the site of the bite, although most cases are demonstrated by antibody testing. The screening ELISA or immuno-fluorescent antibody tests are subject to low sensitivity and low specificity. Acute infection is confirmed by immunoblot assay. Early disease in particular may be 'antibody negative' and a clinical diagnosis is the only method available.
- Non-specific abnormalities include a raised ESR, a high IgM level and abnormally high levels of aminotransferase.
- Lumbar puncture during one of the phases of neurological disease often reveals a CSF lymphocytosis with elevated protein and some-times the presence of antibodies to *Borrelia burgdorferi*.

Treatment

- In stage I disease, tetracycline 4 mg/kg, 6 hourly, for 2–4 weeks is effective. Penicillin V 7 mg/kg, 6 hourly, and erythromycin 4 mg/kg also have their advocates.

- Stage II and III disease is more difficult to treat, significant failure rates having been obtained after optimal therapy. Cefotaxime 15–30 mg/kg, 8 hourly, for 2–3 weeks is most effective, although ceftriaxime (only available in the UK on a named-patient basis) is as good, if not better. High-dose benzylpenicillin and doxycycline can also be effective.
- Some patients, especially those with neurological disease, may remain permanently disabled.

Prevention

- This is centred on avoidance of tick bites.
- In areas of the USA, tick warnings are issued.
- People entering areas where ticks are present should wear thick clothing over their legs, or at least regularly inspect each other for attached ticks, which can bite without causing pain.

Kawasaki disease

Causative agent

- Unknown.

Epidemiology and pathophysiology

- There were 183 classic and 52 atypical cases reported in the UK between 1983 and 1987. More than 41 000 were reported worldwide by 1982.
- A significant proportion of the reported cases in the UK were in people of Oriental and Caribbean origin. The disease is also found in the USA, Canada and elsewhere in Europe.
- Kawasaki disease is also known as mucocutaneous lymph node syndrome. It was first described in Japan in 1969, where it has the highest prevalence; even in America, there is disproportionately high attack rate in Japanese children.
- The peak age of onset is between 18 months and 2 years. It is rare after the age of 5 years, although occasional adult cases have been reported.
- Its importance lies in the high incidence of concomitant coronary artery disease (CAD) as a complication giving rise, in particular, to coronary aneurysms and subsequent rupture, or MI.

Clinical features

● There are six principal symptoms.

1 Fever lasting for 5 days, although the average duration is 7–10 days. There is no response to antibiotics or antipyretics.
2 Non-purulent conjunctivitis: this clears after 1 week.
3 Fissuring, drying out and redness of the lips. The tongue may look like the strawberry tongue of scarlet fever.
4 Lymphadenopathy, which can be generalized but is usually cervical, with large, tender, firm, non-fluctuant glands, often as a single matted group. Lymphadenopathy is the most common of the main symptoms occurring in up to 82% of cases.
5 A morbilliform (measles-like), pleomorphic, rubelliform or erythema multiforme-like rash on the trunk is seen in 99% of cases.
6 Erythema of the hands and feet progressing to indurative oedema, followed by desquamation starting around the finger nails, 10–14 days from the start of the illness.

● As well as the principal symptoms described above, there may be several other associated features, including upper abdominal pain, diarrhoea, arthralgia, mild jaundice, aseptic meningitis and hydrops of the gallbladder.
● The most serious complication is CAD which is detected in 20% of untreated cases.
● Pericarditis, myocarditis, arthritis and urethritis have also been reported.
● The typical disease starts with fever: conjunctivitis, lip and tongue changes, rash, lymphadenopathy and oedematous/erythematous extremities appear within 5 days. Desquamation is seen in the 2nd week, which is when aneurysms may start to develop, although they can occur months later.
● Disease activity can persist 3 or more months.

Differential diagnosis

● The main differential diagnoses are scarlet fever, Stevens–Johnson syndrome, measles, rubella, juvenile rheumatoid arthritis and drug reactions, especially the ampicillin rash seen with EBV infection.

Diagnosis

● Diagnosis is made on clinical criteria: 5 of the 6 principal symptoms (*see* above) must be present.

- Haematological investigations reveal a significant neutrophil leucocytosis, raised ESR, raised CRP and from the 10th day the platelets are elevated, sometimes to $>1000 \times 10^9/l$.
- ECG changes may also occur.
- Ultrasonography is usually adequate to delineate coronary artery size, although angiography may be required.

Treatment

- Aspirin in a dose of 80-100 mg/kg/day, reduced, when the child becomes afebrile, to 3–5 mg/kg/day until the platelet count is normal.
- High-dose iv gammaglobulin (400 mg/kg/day) must be given as early as possible during the first 2 weeks of the illness, as it prevents CAD developing. There is usually an associated rapid defervescence.
- Steroids are contraindicated.
- Careful follow-up with coronary artery scanning is required for up to 1 year after the start of the infection.

Prevention

- Precise preventive measures cannot be taken until the aetiology is defined.

Haemolytic uraemic syndrome (HUS)

Causative agents

- Verotoxigenic *E. coli* usually serotype 0157.
- Imported cases may be caused by *Shigella dysenteriae*.

Epidemiology and pathophysiology

- Occasional sporadic cases or outbreaks are seen in children, usually aged 2–5 years.
- There is a worldwide distribution, although it is especially common in Canada (*E. coli*) and Central and South America (*Shigella*).
- The responsible strains of *E. coli* are mainly food derived. Shigellae are transmitted from person to person by food, water or direct contact.
- There is a peak incidence in July/August. Approximately 120 cases are reported annually in children in the UK.
- Both *E. coli* and *Shigella* produce verocytotoxin.

Incubation period

● 2–7 days.

Clinical features

● The illness in most cases starts with diarrhoea, which may be mild, but is often severe and blood-stained, accompanied by fever and systemic upset.
● Other features of the illness soon develop, including oliguria or anuria and anaemia. In severe cases, purpura, bleeding and focal neurological damage can occur. The mortality rate is 2–10%. Some children are left with renal failure and neurological damage. The rest recover renal function within 4 weeks. Up to 60% of children affected are only mildly affected, and some cases are found incidentally, being without symptoms or signs.
● Thrombotic thrombocytopenic purpura, a similar condition with more neurological damage and seen in older people, may be a variant of HUS.

Differential diagnosis

● The haemorrhagic colitis should be differentiated from other similar diseases including inflammatory bowel disease and other types of gastroenteritis.
● Dehydration, leading to uraemia should be distinguished from the renal failure of this condition.

Diagnosis

● Microangiopathic haemolytic anaemia, and renal dysfunction are the hallmarks of this condition. Thrombocytopenia, leucocytosis and evidence of disseminated intravascular coagulation may be found.
● Culture of organisms (20% are negative).

Treatment

● Maintenance of fluid and electrolyte balance.
● Most cases recover without drug therapy.
● Dialysis is occasionally required for more severe cases, as is blood or platelet transfusion. No other therapy has so far been of proven benefit for all cases.

Prevention

● Good food and water hygiene.

CHAPTER 17

Immunization and preservation of health

ALTHOUGH the decline in incidence of many infectious diseases in the UK this century can largely be ascribed to improving standards of nutrition and hygiene, immunization has also played a part. The eradication of smallpox was undoubtedly due to an effective vaccine and there are other equally powerful vaccines capable of achieving a similar outcome given the commitment and adequate resources.

This chapter is a guide to the various vaccines and immunoglobulins available and their use. More detailed information can be obtained from specialist texts, such as *Immunisation Against Infectious Diseases* (which is regularly updated) published by the DoH, Welsh Office and Scottish Home and Health Department, and supplied free to all doctors. *The Traveller's Guide to Health* (booklet T_1) also published by the DoH provides up-to-date information for travellers.

General considerations

Immunity to an illness can be induced *actively* by injecting the agent in an attenuated or killed form, or one of its antigenically important components. After appropriate immunization, the immunological memory persists for many years and is frequently lifelong. This type of immunity often requires several months before it becomes effective.

Passive immunity is provided by the injection of antibodies known to have specificity for the infectious agent in question. Protection lasts as long as adequate serum levels of antibody are maintained, usually only a matter of weeks. However, immunity begins as soon as the injection is given and may be effective against infective agents acquired within the preceding few days.

Vaccination (a term used interchangeably with active immunization) should be carried out by skilled operators (doctor or nurse), ideally in a setting where the occasional severe reaction, such as anaphylaxis, can be dealt with efficiently. Drugs that are suitable for the treatment of anaphylactic reactions include adrenaline 1 mg/l (1/1000) given im in a dose ranging from 0.05 ml in infants to 1 ml in adults. Steroids, antihistamines and iv fluids can also be useful.

Strict records, including the vaccine batch number, should be kept at each attendance.

The majority of vaccinations are given as deep subcutaneous injections or im. The intradermal route can be used for certain vaccines, including hepatitis B, rabies and typhoid, but should be administered only by a person skilled in this technique. The deltoid area is the preferred site, although the anterior thigh may also be used, especially in infants. The buttocks should not be utilized as the variable fat cover in this region, especially in females, has led to a high failure rate for some vaccines.

Contraindications to immunization

Specific contraindications will be dealt with in the section on individual vaccines, but there are some general rules.

- Vaccination should be temporarily withheld from any patient suffering an acute febrile illness, although minor coryzal symptoms are not included.
- Minor reactions are expected after all vaccines. Only major reactions constitute a contraindication to further doses; these include anaphylaxis and other types of hypersensitivity reaction, severe local reaction (prolonged erythema and induration), convulsions or severe prolonged high fever.
- Live vaccines are usually withheld in pregnancy and the immunocompromised (due to malignancy, steroids, cytotoxics, radiotherapy or HIV infection). There are, however, exceptions to this rule. For instance, pregnant women may receive some live vaccines if their potential disease exposure is high, for instance, when travelling to the tropics. HIV-positive patients whose immune system is still intact may also benefit from some live vaccines. In the case of immunosuppressive drug use, the live vaccines can be given from 6 months after the therapy has ceased. In such cases as these, passive immunization is a good, temporary alternative after disease exposure. Oral polio vaccine should *not* be given to household contacts of the immunocompromised, as this live-attenuated vaccine is readily transmitted from person to person. *NB*: This does not apply to other live vaccines.
- If immunoglobulin preparations are to be given, ideally their administration should be deferred until 3 weeks after a live vaccine has been given. If the immunoglobulin is given first, 3 months should elapse before a live vaccine is given. Possible exceptions to this rule are polio and yellow fever vaccines.
- HIV positive patients may be given all vaccinations *except* polio, BCG and yellow fever.

Table 17.1 The recommended vaccination schedule for children in the UK

Age	Vaccine	Notes
2, 3 and 4 months	Diphtheria/pertussis/tetanus (DPT) plus oral polio vaccine (OPV)	Pertussis can be omitted if specifically contraindicated and diphtheria, tetanus (DT) vaccine substituted
15 months	Mumps, measles, rubella vaccine (MMR)	Introduced 1988. 'Catch-up' vaccination can be given at any time (e.g. pre-school entry)
4–5 years	DPT	Pre-school boosters
10–14 years	Rubella	For girls only; may be phased out when MMR has been extensively used
10–14 years	BCG	Wait 3 weeks between rubella and BCG vaccines. BCG can be given to neonates from ethnic minorities who are at increased risk
15–18 years	Tetanus and OPV	Post-school booster

'Childhood' vaccines

The recommended vaccination schedule for children in the UK is given in Table 17.1. (*See* also General considerations and contraindications, page 203–4.)

Pertussis (whooping cough)

● A killed whole-cell vaccine.
● It is usually given as part of the triple (DPT) vaccine, although a monovalent vaccine is available.
● A newer acellular vaccine is under trial and may be introduced at a later date.

Specific contraindications
● A severe reaction to previous pertussis vaccine, especially fits or prolonged screaming episodes.
● Specialized advice may be sought before vaccinating children with documented previous cerebral damage, known history of convulsions or parents or siblings with epilepsy.

Adverse reactions

● Pain/swelling at the injection site, fever, and screaming episodes.
● Rarely, brain damage and convulsions occur – estimated at approximately 1:100 000 doses, although the actual incidence may be less.

Diphtheria

● A toxoid (altered toxin) vaccine.
● Given as part of the DPT or DT combinations.
● A low-dose vaccine can be given to children over 10 years and adults at risk, for instance, during diphtheria outbreaks, or to certain hospital staff.
● Immunity can be assessed with the Schick test, where intradernal toxoid is injected. Continuing immunity will be shown by a lack of local reaction after 72 hours. If positive (i.e. a reaction occurs), a booster vaccination can be given. This test is still used for high-risk healthcare workers.

Specific contraindications

● A previous severe reaction to the vaccine.

Adverse reactions

● Local pain and swelling, malaise, and fever.
● Very rarely, anaphylaxis and neurological symptoms occur.

Tetanus

● A toxoid vaccine.
● After the pre-school booster, 2 further boosters are recommended at 10-year intervals, following which immunity is assumed to be lifelong.
● Vaccination schedules appropriate for contaminated wounds are recommended in the section on clinical aspects of tetanus (Chapter 14).

Contraindications

● Previous severe reactions only.

Adverse reactions

● Local pain and swelling.
● Rarely, systemic upset or anaphylaxis.
● Persistent induration if the injection is too shallow.

Poliomyelitis

- An oral live attenuated vaccine containing the 3 serotypes. A killed, injectable vaccine is also available.
- Boosters are required at 10-year intervals in adults at continuing risk, such as those who regularly travel in underdeveloped countries. Ideally, the booster should be of the same type of vaccine given for the primary course; if in doubt, give the oral vaccine.
- The injectable vaccine can be given to those unable to tolerate the live vaccine, including the immunocompromised, HIV-positive subjects and women in late pregnancy. However, OPV is probably safe in these groups.
- The OPV can be used during outbreaks of polio due to 'wild' virus.

Contraindications

- For the OPV: intercurrent diarrhoea and vomiting, the immuno-compromised, HIV-positive and pregnant (but see above) and known polymyxin sensitivity.
- *For both vaccines*: previous severe reactions to the vaccine and known sensitivity to streptomycin, neomycin and penicillin.

NB: OPV should be separated from other live vaccines by a 3-week interval unless given simultaneously. Although immunoglobulin may contain antipolio antibodies, its prior administration does not necess-arily prevent the use of OPV.

Adverse reactions

- A vaccine strain-related paralytic illness has occasionally been seen (approximately 2 per 2 million doses).

Measles

- A live-attenuated virus.
- It is most commonly given as part of the MMR vaccine.
- It is not recommended for immunocompromised patients, although it can be used in HIV-positive children. In children unable to receive this vaccine, human normal immunoglobulin has value in providing passive immunity in cases of recent contact.

Specific contraindications

- Pregnancy.
- The immunocompromised.
- A history of severe hypersensitivity following neomycin, polymyxin and eggs.

Adverse reactions

● Fever and malise, sometimes with a rash, are common 5–10 days after vaccination. Parents with children prone to febrile convulsions should be warned of the potential fever.
● Encephalitis is rare.

Mumps, measles, rubella

● Three live-attenuated vaccines are given as a single dose.
● This vaccine has replaced measles monovalent vaccine in most circumstances. The MMR should be given even if the child has previously had measles vaccine or clinical measles.
● The vaccine can be given to HIV-positive children.

Specific contraindications

● The immunocompromised.
● Pregnancy.
● Those who have hypersensitivity reactions to neomycin, kanamycin or eggs.

Adverse reactions

● As for measles vaccine.
● Parotid swelling and aseptic meningitis may also follow.

Tuberculosis (Bacillus Calmette-Guérin)

● A live-attenuated vaccine.
● Usually given as an intradermal injection of 0.1 ml in adults, or 0.05 ml in infants of ethnic minorities. Although the deltoid is normally used in adults, the sole of the foot may be utilized in infants, because it leaves a less unsightly scar.

Assessment of immunity

● Immunity is normally assessed initially with the Mantoux test or Heaf test.

1 In Mantoux testing, an intradermal injection of 0.1 ml purified protein derivative (ppd) containing 10 tuberculin units (1/1000) or 100 iu (1/100), is given and the resulting induration measured at 72–96 hours.

2 The Heaf test is more suitable for mass testing but has the disadvantage of requiring re-usable apparatus which must be sterilized. 100 000 units/ml of ppd is applied to an area of skin and 6 needles passed through this into the skin at a depth of 2 mm (1 mm in infants). Induration is assessed at 3-10 days.

Interpretation of Mantoux and Heaf tests

For interpretation of the tests, *see* Table 17.2.

Table 17.2 Interpretation of Mantoux and Heaf tests

Mantoux (10 tu, 1/1000) Reaction (Induration)	Heaf test	Interpretation
0–5 mm	*Heaf 0:* No, or faint reaction	Non-immune
6–10 mm	*Heaf 1:* At least 4 indurated papules	Past BCG or atypical mycobacterial infection
11–15 mm	*Heaf 2:* Confluent papules in an indurated ring	As above, or past TB
16+ mm	*Heaf 3:* Induration of 5–10 mm *Heaf 4:* >10 mm induration	As above, but is suspicious of active TB

- Adults or children with a reaction equivalent to Heaf 0 should be revaccinated if BCG was previously given, unless there is a scar that demonstrates a successful initial vaccination. If BCG has been previously administered, a reaction of Heaf 1 or greater indicates successful vaccination.
- If BCG has not been given before, vaccination is required for those with Heaf 0 or 1 only. A reaction equivalent to Heaf 3 or Heaf 4 cannot be explained by BCG alone, and recent exposure to, or infection with, TB should be considered.
- Adults who should be assessed for immunity include health service staff, TB contacts and travellers intending to spend a prolonged time in countries where there is a high prevalence of TB.

Specific contraindications
- The immunocompromised.
- Pregnancy.
- HIV-positive subjects.
- Skin sepsis.

Adverse reactions

- Ulceration at the site of injection is common, although occasionally very severe local reactions may require isoniazid therapy.
- Lymphadenitis is common.
- Anaphylaxis is a rare adverse reaction.

Rubella

- A live-attenuated vaccine.
- Rubella vaccine is still given to teenage girls, but vaccination policy is aimed at the eradication of rubella infection in the UK by universal vaccination of young children. When these children reach the teenage years, rubella vaccine may be withdrawn, except for women shown to be non-immune.
- Immunity to rubella infection will continue to be assessed in women of fertile years, ideally before the first pregnancy.
- If anti-D antibody is given to Rhesus-negative women after pregnancy, rubella vaccination can be administered at the same time. The vaccine should not be given during pregnancy.

Specific contraindications

- Pregnancy.
- The immunocompromised.

  Contraception for up to 3 months is recommended following vaccination of adult women.

Adverse reactions

- A mild rubella-like illness may be seen after 1–3 weeks.
- Neurological reactions are rare.

Protecting the traveller: general considerations

Although vaccinating the traveller is important, it is only one aspect of the preparation of individuals before their journey. Advice should be given in the following areas.

1 Food and water hygiene. The only safe drinks are boiled water, pasteurized milk and drinks in sealed bottles or cans. Filtered and halogenated (iodine or chlorine) water is a good second best. Food is safe if thoroughly cooked, or comes in a peel which can then be removed. Salads and cold meats are potentially infective. Freshwater rivers and lakes should not be swum or waded in.

2 Avoidance of bites from insects, especially mosquitoes. This can be achieved by avoiding skin exposure outdoors at dawn and dusk, the use of insect repellants, such as DEET, mosquito meshing on doors and windows, air conditioning, knockdown insecticides contained in burning coils or pads on electric heaters, and mosquito nets impregnated with insect repellant which are inspected frequently.

3 Vaccination and antimalarial regimen. Advice changes frequently and up-to-date information should be sought from a variety of sources including regularly revised publications, specialist vaccination clinics, departments of infectious and tropical diseases, the DoH (071 407 5522), the Communicable Disease Surveillance Centre (081 200 6868) and Communicable Disease (Scotland) Unit (041 946 7120). Accelerated vaccination programmes are available for people who need to travel at short notice.

Travel kits, which contain needles, syringes, sutures, giving sets, blood substitutes and dressings can be purchased from many pharmacists for travellers visiting less developed areas. A covering letter explaining its use from a doctor is advisable for customs and immigration use.

The vaccines listed above, especially polio, tetanus and BCG, should also be considered for adults travelling abroad.

Protecting the traveller: specific vaccines

Cholera

- A killed vaccine.
- It is currently required for entry to Angola, Bangladesh, Cameroon, India, Lesotho, Madagascar, Nigeria, Pakistan, Pitcairn Islands, Somalia, Sudan, Tanzania and Vietnam, although this should be confirmed with the embassy at the time of travel.
- Most authorities regard this vaccination as being of such poor efficacy that its routine use should be discontinued.
- Primary immunization is by 2 subcutaneous or im injections of 0.5–1 ml of vaccine (for the adult) separated by 1–4 weeks. Boosters are required after 6 months, as is a new certificate of vaccination.

Specific contraindications

- Pregnancy.
- Children below 1 year of age.

Adverse reactions
- Local pain and redness, fever and malaise.

Typhoid

- A killed vaccine.
- It is recommended for all travellers outside North America, Europe, Australia and New Zealand.
- Primary vaccination consists of 2 doses of 0.5 ml (subcutaneous or im) separated by 4–6 weeks, which lasts for 3 years. A single dose provides 1 year's immunity.

Specific contraindications
- Pregnancy.
- Children under 1 year of age.

Adverse reactions
- Swelling, pain and redness, headache, nausea and fever.

Yellow fever

- A live-attenuated vaccine.
- It can be given only at World Health Organization (WHO) designated vaccination centres.
- After a single dose immunity (and the certificate) lasts for 10 years. The certificate is valid only after 10 days have elapsed following vaccination.

Specific contraindications
- Pregnancy.
- HIV-positive subjects.
- The immunocompromised.
- Infants below 9 months.
- Hypersensitivity to eggs, neomycin or polymyxin.

NB: Human normal immunoglobulin does not interfere with this vaccination.

Adverse reactions
- Local pain, headache, fever and myalgia.

Hepatitis B

- A genetically engineered or plasma-derived viral component (surface protein).
- 3 doses at 0, 1 and 6 months are recommended, although a rapid course of 0, 1 and 2 months gives good results.
- A protection rate of 90% is achieved, failures being most frequent in subjects who are over 45 years of age, fat or female. The duration of protection varies widely, but on average it is 3 years.
- The disease is endemic throughout the tropics and subtropics, especially South East Asia. Vaccination should be offered to health personnel both in this country and if travelling abroad. Long-term travellers may also be considered.
- Hepatitis B-specific immunoglobulin is available for patients at risk (e.g. needlestick) (see below).

Specific contraindications
- None.

Adverse reactions
- Local pain and swelling only.

Rabies

- A killed virus vaccine (derived from human diploid cells).
- Rabies is endemic in much of the world, although the majority of cases seen in the UK are acquired in India.
- A primary course consists of 2 doses of 1 ml subcutaneous or im given at a 4-week interval. For post-exposure vaccination see the section on rabies in Chapter 14 (page 170).
- Boosters are required every 1–3 years depending on risk – mainly recommended for veterinary surgeons and long-term visitors to the Indian subcontinent.

Specific contraindications
- Hypersensitivity to a preceding dose.
- Pregnancy (except if risk of exposure is high).

Adverse reactions
- Local pain and swelling.
- Fever, headache, myalgia, vomiting and urticaria.
- Rarely, anaphylaxis and Guillain–Barré syndrome.

Meningococcal vaccine (A and C types)

- A killed vaccine.
- It is effective only against epidemic strains A and C, which are seen most frequently in the meningitis belt of subsaharan Africa (15°N to 5°N plus Uganda and Kenya to the equator), in the dry season. Also in Saudi Arabia, the New Delhi area and Nepal.
- A single dose (0.5 ml, subcutaneous or im) provides 3 years' immunity.

Specific contraindications

- Children <2 months of age.

Adverse reactions

- Local pain and tenderness and fever.

Japanese B encephalitis

- A killed virus vaccine.
- An endemic disease in rural South East Asia and the Far East during the monsoon, transmitted by the bites of culicine mosquitoes from infected pigs.
- Recommended for long-term travellers in rural areas during the rainy season.
- Primary vaccination is two 1 ml injections, subcutaneous or im, given 7–14 days apart. Boosters are required every year. A primary course of three injections with the third a further month after the initial two provides a rapid, higher rate of protection.

Specific contraindications

- Fever.
- Severe systemic illness.
- Diabetes.
- Leukaemia.
- Lymphoma.
- Other malignancies.
- Known hypersensitivity.
- Pregnancy.

Adverse reactions

- Local pain and swelling.
- Fever.

Tick-borne encephalitis

- A killed vaccine.
- This disease is endemic in rural forest areas of central Europe and Scandinavia in the summer.
- The infection is transmitted from infected animals by tick bites which should be avoided (*see* Lyme disease, page 197).
- Three 0.5 ml injections, subcutaneous or im, at 0, 1 and 4 months form the primary course. Boosters are required after 3 years.

Specific contraindications

- Fever.
- Allergy to egg.

Adverse reactions

- Local pain and swelling.
- Fever.

Malaria prophylaxis

- Deaths due to falciparum malaria in travellers are still common.
- Measures to avoid mosquito bites (page 162) are very important.
- Drug prophylaxis should start 1 week before the journey and continue until 4 weeks after return.
- The extent of the geographical spread of drug-resistant malaria is changing rapidly and up to date information should be sought from weekly publications (e.g. *Pulse*), specialist vaccination clinics, Communicable Disease Surveillance Centre (*see* page 178 for details).
- Current recommendations include proguanil 200 mg daily and chloroquine 300 mg base weekly (in adults) for most areas endemic for malaria, with Maloprim weekly as an alternative to the proguanil. The Maloprim regimen is recomended for those visiting Papua New Guinea, Solomon Islands and Vanuatu.
- Prophylaxis may fail even when taken regularly, but especially if the drugs are not absorbed due to diarrhoea or vomiting.

Human normal immunoglobulin (for hepatitis A prevention)

- This is given to young adults at risk of catching hepatitis A, such as visitors to the tropics and subtropics.

- It should be given a few days before travel to provide maximum efficacy and to avoid interference with the effect of live vaccines (*see* page 204).
- A dose of 250–500 mg (in adults) gives 3–6 months' protection.
- It can also be used for post-exposure prophylaxis.

Specific contraindications
- None.

NB: It should not be given 3 months before or 3 weeks after most live vaccines.

Adverse reactions
- Generally mild.
- Anaphylaxis has been rarely reported.

Other vaccines

Influenza

- A killed virus vaccine.
- The antigenic content is changed yearly in response to the expected epidemic strains (usually of types A and B).
- Vaccination is required annually with a dose of 0.5 ml, subcutaneous or im in at-risk groups, such as those with chronic heart, lung or kidney disease, diabetics, and the elderly, institutionalized and immunocompromised.

Specific contraindications
- Egg allergy.
- Children <4 years of age.

Adverse reactions
- Local reactions.
- 'Flu-like illness.
- Hypersensitivity (rare).

Pneumococcal vaccine

- A killed vaccine.
- Recommended prior to splenectomy or in some patients with chronic heart or lung disease.

- A single 0.5 ml injection, subcutaneous or im, is recommended. Boosters can be given only after 5 years.

Specific contraindications
- Hypersensitivity to previous doses.
- Pregnancy and breast feeding.
- Children <2 years of age.

Anthrax

- Recommended for workers exposed to disease.
- 4 injections at 3 weekly intervals between first 3 and 6 months between third and fourth annual boosters.

Passive immunity

Human normal immunoglobulin (*see* also above)

- It can be given as pre- or post-exposure prophylaxis for hepatitis A.
- It might also prevent measles if given soon after exposure.
- Although there is some anti-rubella and anti-mumps specificity, it should not be relied upon to prevent these conditions.

Hepatitis B specific immunoglobulin

- This can be given to the non-immune with tetanus-prone wounds (*see* section on tetanus, Chapter 14 page 173).
- Effective if given within 48 hours after parenteral or sexual exposure to hepatitis B.

Anti-varicella-zoster immunoglobulin

- This is in short supply but can be given to contacts of chickenpox or shingles, who are immunocompromised or pregnant, and neonates, including those born within 1 week of maternal chickenpox.

Anti-diphtheria and anti-botulism immunoglobulins

- These are available for the rare circumstance of clinical disease.

Anti-tetanus immunoglobulin

- For treatment of tetanus prone wounds in the unimmunized; those whose immunization history is unknown and those who have not had a booster in 10 years.

Sources of vaccines and immunoglobulins

- *Most* vaccines can be obtained through the usual pharmaceutical outlets.
- Yellow fever vaccine can be administered only at designated centres, a list of which is available from the DoH.
- Rabies vaccine for pre-exposure vaccinations can be ordered from Merieux (UK) Ltd (0628 78529). Post-exposure vaccination and human rabies immunoglobulin can be obtained quickly via the Public Health Laboratory Service (PHLS) Virus Reference Laboratory (081 200 4400) or in Scotland via the Communicable Disease (Scotland) Unit (041 946 7120) and the regional infectious diseases units.
- Meningococcal vaccine can be obtained from most travel clinics and vaccine suppliers for pre-exposure vaccinations. In outbreaks due to types A or C in closed institutions, or close contacts of index cases due to these strains, post-exposure vaccination can be administered after discussion with the Communicable Disease Surveillance Centre (081 200 6868) or (041 946 7120) and the Meningococcal Reference Laboratories – England and Wales: 061 445 2416; Scotland: 041 946 7120.
- Japanese B encephalitis vaccination may be obtained from some travel clinics or ordered from the suppliers (091 261 5950). Tick-borne encephalitis vaccine can be obtained in the same way (0732 458101).
- Human normal immunoglobulin can be obtained commercially or, in emergencies, via the PHLS (081 200 6868), the Blood Transfusion Service (Scotland) or the laboratories, Belfast City Hospital (0232 329341). Information on supplies of anti-tetanus, anti-hepatitis B and anti-zoster immunoglobulins can also be obtained from these sources.

Appendix 1 Notifiable diseases

THE Health Service and Public Health Act 1968 requires that a doctor must notify the local Communicable Disease Centre (formerly the Medical Officer for Environmental Health) of a patient with any of the following infectious diseases. A fee is payable for each notification.

Anthrax
Cholera
Diphtheria
Dysentery (amoebic or bacillary)
Encephalitis (acute)
Food poisoning (actual or suspected)
Hepatitis
Infective jaundice
Lassa fever
Leprosy
Leptospirosis
Malaria
Marburg disease
Measles
Meningitis
Meningococcal septicaemia
Mumps
Ophthalmia neonatorum
Paratyphoid fever A or B
Plague
Poliomyelitis
Rabies
Relapsing fever
Rubella
Scarlet fever
Tetanus
Tuberculosis (all forms)
Typhoid fever
Typhus fever
Viral haemorrhagic fever
Whooping cough
Yellow fever

In Scotland notification is to the Chief Administrative Medical Officer, and the list does not include:

Encephalitis
Infective jaundice
Tetanus
Tuberculosis

but does include:

Continued fever
Erysipelas
Leptospiral jaundice
Membranous croup
Puerperal fever
Viral hepatitis

In Northern Ireland notification is to the Chief Administrative Medical Officer, and the list does not include:

Food poisoning
Infective jaundice
Leprosy
Malaria

but does include:

Gastroenteritis (if under 2 years old)
Infective hepatitis

AIDS is not notifiable but can be voluntarily registered at the Communicable Disease Surveillance Centre, 61 Colindale Avenue, London NW9 5EQ (081 200 6868) or in Scotland the Communicable Disease Unit, Ruchill Hospital, Glasgow G20 9NB (041 9467 7120).

Toxic shock syndrome is not notifiable although reporting to the local Public Health Laboratory is recommended.

Appendix 2 Incubation periods of some infectious diseases

THE incubation period is the interval between the time of primary infection or contact with an infected person, and the appearance of the disease. These are meant only as a guide because rare cases of several of these diseases have been recognized which have had an incubation period outside that of the stated range.

Disease or causative organism	Incubation period
Amoebic dysentery	1–4 weeks
Amoebic liver abscess	2 weeks to several years
Bacillus cereus enteritis	1–5 hours
Botulism	2 hours to 8 days, usually 12–36 hours
Brucellosis	1–8 weeks, usually 2–3 weeks
Campylobacter enteritis	1–11 days, usually 2–5 days
Chickenpox	10–21 days, usually 14–15 days
Cholera	2–48 hours
Clostridium perfingens-toxin enteritis	8–22 hours
Dysentery, *Shigella*	1–7 days, usually 1–3 days
Infective jaundice (hepatitis A)	14–42 days
Hepatitis B	42 days to 6 months
Influenza	1–5 days
Lassa fever	3–17 days
Legionnaires' disease	2–10 days
Leptospirosis	4–19 days, usually 7–12 days
Malaria	8–25 days, but relapse/recrudescence may be seen up to many years later
Marburg virus disease	3–9 days
Measles	7–21 days, usually 10–14 days
Mumps	12–28 days, usually 16–18 days
Polio	10–15 days
Q fever	9–20 days
Rabies	2 weeks to 5 years, usually 20–90 days
Rubella	14–21 days, usually 18 days
Salmonella enteritis	6–72 hours
Scarlet fever	2–5 days
Syphilis (primary)	9–90 days
Tick typhus	7–18 days
Typhoid fever	7–21 days
Whooping cough	5–21 days
Yellow fever	3–6 days

Appendix 3 Vaccinations for foreign travel

Country	Cholera[9]	Malaria*	Typhoid	Polio	Yellow fever
Afghanistan[6]	●	C[4]	●	●	▼
Albania	5		●	●	▼
Algeria			●	●	▼
Angola	●	A	●	●	●[1]▼
Antilles, Netherlands			●	●	▼
Argentina		A	●	●	
Azores			●	●	▼
Bahamas			●	●	▼
Bahrain			●	●	
Bangladesh[6]	●	A	●	●	▼
Barbados			●	●	▼
Belize		C	●	●	▼
Benin[6]	●	A	●	●	●[1]
Bhutan	●	A	●	●	▼
Bolivia		A	●	●	●[1]▼
Botswana		A[4]	●	●	
Brazil		A[7]	●	●	●[1]▼
Brunei	●		●	●	▼
Burkino Faso	●	A	●	●	●[1]
Burundi	●	A	●	●	●[1]▼
Cameroon[6]	●	A[7]	●	●	●[1]
Canal Zone, Panama		A	●	●	
Cape Verde Islands		C	●	●	▼
Cayman Islands			●	●	
Central African Rep.	●	A	●	●	●[1]
Chad[6]	●	A	●	●	●[1]▼
Chile			●	●	
China		A[7,8]	●	●	▼
Colombia		A	●	●	●[1]▼
Comoros			●	●	
Congo	●	A	●	●	●[1]
Cook Islands			●	●	
Costa Rica		C	●	●	
Cuba			●	●	
Djibouti	●	A	●	●	▼
Dominica			●	●	▼
Dominican Republic		C	●	●	
Ecuador		A	●	●	●[1]
Egypt		C[4,8]	●	●	▼
El Salvador		C	●	●	▼
Equatorial Guinea	●	A	●	●	●[1]▼
Ethiopia[6]	●	A	●	●	▼

Country	Cholera[9]	Malaria*	Typhoid	Polio	Yellow fever
Fiji			●	●	
Gabon[6]	●	A	●	●	●[1]
Gambia	●	A	●	●	●[1]
Grenada			●	●	▼
Guam			●	●	▼
Guatemala		C	●	●	▼
Guiana, French		A	●	●	●[1]
Guinea[6]	●	A	●	●	●[1]▼
Guinea Bissau[6]	●	A	●	●	●[1]▼
Guyana		A	●	●	●[1]
Haiti		C	●	●	▼
Honduras		C	●	●	▼
Hong Kong			●	●	
India[6]	●[2]	A	●	●	▼
Indonesia[6]		A[7]	●	●	▼
Iran		A[4]	●	●	▼
Iraq		C[4]	●	●	▼
Israel			●	●	
Ivory Coast[6]	●	A	●	●	●[1]
Jamaica			●	●	▼
Jordan			●	●	
Kampuchea	●	A[7]	●	●	
Kenya[6]	[5]	A[7]	●	●	●[1]▼
Kiribati			●	●	▼
Korea (North)			●	●	
Korea (South)			●	●	
Kuwait			●	●	
Laos (Lao)	●	A[7]	●	●	▼
Lebanon	●		●	●	▼
Lesotho	●		●	●	▼
Liberia[6]	●	A	●	●	●[1]
Libya		C[4]	●	●	▼
Madagascar	●[5]	A	●		▼
Madeira				●	▼
Malawi	●	A[7]	●	●	▼
Malaysia		A	●	●	▼
Maldives			●	●	▼
Mali	●	A	●	●	●[1]
Malta	[5]			●	▼
Mauritania	●	C	●	●	●[1]
Mauritius		C	●	●	▼
Mexico		C	●	●	▼
Mongolia			●	●	
Montserrat			●	●	▼
Morocco			●	●	
Mozambique	●	A	●	●	▼
Myanmar (Burma)	●	A[7]	●	●	▼
Namibia	●	A	●	●	●▼
Nauru			●	●	▼
Nepal[6]	●	A	●	●	▼

Country	Cholera[9]	Malaria*	Typhoid	Polio	Yellow fever
New Caledonia	5		●	●	▼
Nicaragua		C	●	●	▼
Niger	●	A	●	●	●[1]
Nigeria[6]	●	A	●	●	●
Niue			●	●	▼
Oman		C	●	●	▼
Pakistan[6]	●[5]	A	●	●	▼
Panama		A	●	●	●[1]
Papua New Guinea	●[1]	B[7]	●	●	▼
Paraguay		C	●	●	▼
Peru		C	●	●	●[1]▼
Philippines		A[7]	●	●	▼
Pitcairn Island	5		●	●	
Polynesia, French			●	●	▼
Puerto Rico			●	●	
Qatar			●	●	▼
Reunion Islands			●	●	▼
Rwanda	●	A	●	●	●[1]▼
Saint Helena			●	●	
Saint Lucia			●	●	▼
Saint Vincent and Grenadines			●	●	▼
Samoa			●	●	▼
Sao Tomé and Principe	●	A	●	●	●[1]▼
Saudi Arabia[6]		C[4]	●	●	▼
Senegal[6]	●	A	●	●	●
Seychelles			●	●	
Sierra Leone[6]	●	A	●	●	●[1]
Singapore			●	●	▼
Solomon Islands		B[7]	●	●	▼
Somalia[6]	●	A	●	●	●[1]▼
South Africa		A[4]	●	●	▼
Sri Lanka	●	A	●	●	▼
Sudan[6]	●[5]	A	●	●	●[1]▼
Surinam		A	●	●	●[1]▼
Swaziland	●[5]	A	●	●	▼
Syria		C[4]	●	●	▼
Taiwan			●	●	
Tanzania[6]	●[3]	A	●	●	●[1]▼
Thailand		A[7]	●	●	▼
Timor, East			●	●	●
Togo[6]		A	●	●	●[1]▼
Trinidad and Tobago			●	●	▼
Tunisia			●	●	▼
Turkey		C[4]	●	●	
Tuvalu			●	●	▼
Uganda[6]	●	A[7]	●	●	●[1]
United Arab Emirates		C[4]	●	●	▼
Uruguay			●	●	
Vanuatu		B[7]	●	●	

Country	Cholera[9]	Malaria*	Typhoid	Polio	Yellow fever
Venezuela		A[4]	●	●	●[1]
Vietnam		A[7]	●	●	
Virgin Islands			●	●	
West Indies Associated States			●	●	
West Indies, French			●	●	▼
Yemen Arab Republic[6] (North)	●[5]	A[4]	●	●	▼
Yemen Rep (South)[6]	●	C	●	●	▼
Zaire[6]	●	A[7]	●	●	●
Zambia	●	A[7]	●	●	●[1]▼
Zimbabwe		A	●	●	▼

● Vaccinations that are an essential requirement.
● Vaccinations or tablets that are recommended for protection against disease.
No prophylactic vaccinations or tablets are necessary for countries that are not listed.
[1] Except children under one year old.
[2] A certificate may be required on leaving.
[3] Compulsory if visiting Zanzibar or Pemba.
[4] Seasonal risk.
[5] Compulsory if crossing an infected area within 6 days.
[6] *Meningitis A* and C vaccination recommended particularly for travellers in rural areas; vaccination should be given at least 10 days before departure.
[7] Mefloquine should be considered for high-risk short-term stay (1 to 3 weeks): 1 tablet weekly for 6 weeks starting the week before travel.
[8] Not generally needed for tourist trips.
[9] Cholera vaccine is of low efficacy and use is declining. A single dose is adequate to satisfy certification requirements.
▼ A certificate may be required for travellers crossing *yellow fever* areas.
* Recommendations correct at time of going to press: first check with Malaria Reference Laboratory (071 636 7921) 24-hour taped advice or ring 071 636 8636 9am to 3pm Monday to Friday. Area A proguanil (Paludrine) 200 mg daily, plus chloroquine (Avloclor, Nivaquine) 300 mg base weekly. Area B Maloprim one tablet weekly, chloroquine 300 mg base weekly. Area C proguanil 200 mg daily or chloroquine 300 mg base weekly. If travelling to remote areas *typhoid, hepatitis A, polio, tetanus, rabies* and *Japanese B encephalitis* injections should also be considered.

Glossary

AV	Atrioventricular
AIDS	Acquired Immune Deficiency Syndrome
ALT	Alanine Transferase
ANUG	Acute Necrotizing Ulcerative Gingivitis
ARC	AIDS Related Complex
ASO	Antistreptolypsin O
AZT	Azidothymidine
BCG	Bacillus Calmette Guérin
CAD	Coronary Artery Disease
CCDC	Consultant in Communicable Disease Control
CDC	Center for Disease Control
CMV	Cytomegalovirus
CNS	Central Nervous System
CRP	C Reactive Protein
CSF	Cerebrospinal Fluid
CT	Computerized Tomography
CVA	Cerebrovascular Accident
DEAFF	Detection of Early Antigen by Fluorescent Foci
DEET	Diethyltoluamide
DHF	Dengue Haemorrhagic Fever
DNA	Deoxyribonucleic Acid
DoH	Department of Health
DPT	Diphtheria, Pertussis, Tetanus
DT	Diphtheria, Tetanus
EA	Early Antigen
EBNA	Epstein–Barr Nuclear Antigen
EBV	Epstein–Barr Virus
ECG	Electrocardiogram
ECHO	Enterocytopathogenic Human Orphan
ECHO	Echoencephalogram
ECM	Erythema Chronicum Migrans
EDTA	Ethylenediaminetetra-acetic Acid
EEG	Electroencephalography
EIEC	Entero-invasive E. coli
ELISA	Enzyme Linked Immunoadsorbent Assay
EM	Erythema multiforme
EPEC	Enteropathogenic E. coli
ESR	Erythrocyte Sedimentation Rate

ETEC	Enterotoxigenic *E. coli*
FTA ABS	Fluorescent Treponemal Antibody Absorption Test
GP	General Practitioner
HBeAG	Hepatitis B 'e' Antigen
HBsAG	Hepatitis B Surface Antigen
HHV-6	Human Herpes Virus Type 6
HIV	Human Immunodeficiency Virus
HSV	Herpes Simplex Virus
HUS	Haemolytic Uraemic Syndrome
IHD	Ischaemic Heart Disease
im	Intramuscular
iv	Intravenous
LFT	Liver Function Test
LGV	Lymphogranuloma Venereum
MAI	Mycobacterium Avium Intracellulare
MI	Myocardial Infarction
MMR	Measles, Mumps & Rubella
MRSA	Methicillin Resistant Staph. Aureus
MSU	Mid-stream Urine Specimen
NGU	Non-gonococcal Urethritis
NSAID	Non-steroidal Anti-inflammatory Drug
OPV	Oral Polio Virus
PCP	Pneumocystis Carinii Pneumonitis
PHLS	Public Health Laboratory Service
PID	Pelvic Inflammatory Disease
PML	Progressive Multifocal Leucoencephalopathy
ppd	Purified Protein Derivative
PUO	Pyrexia of Unknown Origin
RNA	Ribonucleic Acid
RPR	Rapid Plasma Reagin
RSV	Respiratory Syncytial Virus
SRSV	Small Round Structured Virus
STD	Sexually Transmitted Disease
TB	Tuberculosis
TEN	Toxic Epidermal Necrolysis
TPHA	Treponema Pallidum Haemagglutination Assay
TSST-1	Toxic Shock Syndrome Toxin Type I
UK	United Kingdom
UTI	Urinary Tract Infection
UV	Ultraviolet
VCA	Viral Capsular Antigen
VDRL	Venereal Disease Reference Laboratory
VHF	Viral Haemorrhagic Fever
VTEC	Vero-toxin producing *E. coli*

WHO	World Health Organization
^{14}C	Radioactive carbon
°C	Centigrade scale
CO_2	Carbon dioxide
g	Gram
H_2O	Water
iu	International Units
kg	Kilogram
m	metre
M	Mega
mm^3	Millimetres cubed
mg	Milligram
O_2	Oxygen
>	More than
<	Less than
%	Percentage

Reading list

Reference books on infectious and tropical diseases

Christie AB. (1987) *Infectious Diseases*, 4th Edition. Churchill Livingstone, London.

Mandell GL, Douglas RG, Bennett JE (eds). (1990) *Principles and Practice of Infectious Diseases*, 3rd Edition. Churchill Livingstone, London.

Strickland GT. (1984) *Hunters Tropical Medicine*, 6th Edition. WB Saunders, London.

Colour atlases

Emond RTD, Rowland HK. (1987) *A Colour Atlas of Infectious Diseases*. Wolfe Medical Publications, London.

Peters W, Gilles HM. (1989) *A Colour Atlas of Tropical Medicine and Parasitology*. Wolfe Medical Publications, London.

Emond RTD, Bradley JM, Galbraith NS. (1989) *Infection – Pocket Consultant*, 2nd Edition. Blackwell Scientific Publications, Oxford.

Further reading on specific topics covered in the book

Parker DJP, Rose G. (1990) *Epidemiology in Medical Practice*, Churchill Livingstone, Edinburgh.

Skinner C. (1990) Control and Prevention of Tuberculosis in Britain. *Br Med J* **300**:995.

O'Mahony MC, Stanwell Smith RE, Tillett HE. (1990) The Stafford Outbreak of Legionnaires' Disease, *Epidemiol Infection* **104**:361.

Walton W. (1985) *Brain's Diseases of the Nervous System*. Oxford University Press, Oxford.

Parsons M. (1988) *Tuberculous Meningitis*. Oxford Medical Publications, Oxford.

Young SH. (1983) Brain Abscess. A Review of 300 Cases. *J Neurosurg* **59**:735.

Gwalting JM. (1980) Epidemiology of the Common Cold. *Ann NY Acad Sci* **353**:54.

McMillan JA, Sandstrom C, Weiner LB *et al.* (1986) Viral and Bacterial Organisms Associated with Acute Pharyngitis in a School Aged Population. *J Pediatr* **109**:747.

Henderson FW, Collier AM, Sanyal MA. (1982) A Longitudinal Study of Respiratory Viruses and Bacteria in the Aetiology of Acute Otitis Media with Effusion. *N Engl J Med* **306**:1377.

Macfarlane JT, Finch RG. (1982) Hospital Study of Adult Community Acquired Pneumonia. *Lancet* **ii**:255.

Wohl MEB. (1986) Bronchiolitis. *Paediatric Ann* **15**:307.

Seaton A, Seaton D, Leitch AG. (1989) *Crofton and Douglas's Respiratory Diseases*, 4th Edition. Blackwell Scientific Publications, Oxford.

Washington JA. (1987) The Microbiological Diagnosis of Infective Endocarditis. *J Antimicrob Chemother* **20** suppl A:29.

Gorbach SL. (1986) *Infectious Diarrhea*. Blackwell Scientific Publications, Oxford.

Levine MA. (1987) *Escherichia coli* that Cause Diarrhoea. *J Infect Dis* **155**:1377.

Schiff L, Schiff ER. (1987) *Diseases of the Liver*. JB Lippincott, London.

Anon. (1990) Hepatitis C Virus Upstanding. *Lancet* **335**:431.

Choo QL, Kuo G, Weisner AJ *et al.* (1989) Isolation of a C-DNA Clone Derived from a Blood-borne non A non B Viral Hepatitis Genome. *Science* **244**:359.

Zuckerman AJ. (1990) Hepatitis E Virus. *Br Med J* **300**:1475.

Berman SJ, Tsai C, Holmes K *et al.* (1973) Sporadic Anicteric Leptospirosis in South Vietnam. A study of 150 patients. *Ann Intern Med* **79**:167.

Wisdom A. (1988) *A Colour Atlas of Venereology*. Wolfe Medical Books, London.

Adler MW. (1988) *ABC of Sexually Transmitted Diseases*. BMA Publications, London.

Csonka GW, Oates JK. (1990) *Sexually Transmitted Diseases*. Baillière-Tindall, London.

Johnson J, Stamm W. (1987) Diagnosis and Treatment of Acute Urinary Tract Infection. *Infect Dis Clin North Am* **1**:773.

Rubin RH, Tolkoff-Rubin NE, Contrais RB. (1986) Urinary Tract Infection. In: *The Kidney*. Brenner BN, Recton FC, eds. WB Saunders, London 1085.

du Vivier A. (1986) *Atlas of Clinical Dermatology*. Churchill Livingstone, Edinburgh.

Schafrer LA, Taplin D, Scott G, Petal A. (1983) A Therapeutic Update of Superficial Skin Infections. *Paediatr Clin North Am* **30**:397.

Miller SJH. (1989) *Parson's Diseases of the Eye*. Churchill Livingstone, Edinburgh.

Seal DV, Barrett SP, McGill JI. (1982) Aetiology and Treatment of Acute Bacterial Infection of the External Eye. *Br J Ophthalmol* **66**:357.

Anon. (1989) Risks Associated with Human Parvovirus B19 Infection. *J Am Med Assoc* **261**:1406 and 1555.

Yamanishi K, Okuno T, Skiraki K *et al.* (1988) Identification of Human Herpes Virus-6 as a Causal Agent for Exanthem Subitum. *Lancet* **i**:1065.

McCarty DJ. (1989) Infectious Arthritis. In: *Arthritis and Allied Conditions*, pp. 1863–98. Lea and Febger, Philadelphia.

Anon. (1987) Revision of Case Definition for AIDS for Surveillance Purposes. *MMWR* **36**:45.

Sande MA, Volberding PA. (1990) *The Medical Management of AIDS*. WB Saunders, London.

Fischl MA, Richman DD, Greico MH. (1987) The Efficacy of Azidothymidine (AZT) in the Treatment of Patients with AIDS and AIDS-related Complex: a doubleblind, placebo controlled trial. *N Engl J Med* **317**:185.

Manson-Bahr C, Bell DR. (1989) *Manson's Tropical Diseases*. Baillière-Tindall, London.

Hunt JL (ed). (1988) Imported Diseases: a symposium. *Prescriber's Journal* 28.

Warrel DA, Molyneux ME, Beales PF. (1990) Severe and Complicated Malaria. *Trans R Soc Trop Med Hyg* **84**:Suppl 2.

Cook, GO. (1990) Toxoplasma-gondii Infection. *Q J Med* **74**:3.

Steere AC. (1989) Lyme Disease. *N Engl J Med* **321**:586.

Department of Health, Welsh Office, Scottish Home and Health Office. (1990) *Immunization Against Infectious Diseases*. HMSO, London.

Department of Health. (1990) *The Travellers Guide to Health* (leaflet T$_1$). HMSO, London.

Various authors. Modern Vaccines. Weekly from February 24–June 16. *Lancet* 1990:**335**.

Phillips-Howard PA, Radalowicz A, Mitchell J, Bradley DJ. (1990) Risks of Malaria in British Residents Returning from Malarious Areas. *Br Med J* **300**:499.

Index

abscess
  amoebic liver 155, 156
  cerebral 5–6
  pulmonary 38–40
acute bacterial meningitis 5, 7–9
acute necrotizing ulcerative gingivitis
    19–20
acute renal failure 163
African tick typhus 155
AIDS *see* human immunodeficiency
    virus infection
Akureyri disease 194–6
algid malaria 163
amoebic dysentery 158, 159
amoebic liver abscess 155, 156
animals, infections from 2–3
anthrax 217
anti-botulism immunoglobulin 217
anti-diphtheria immunoglobulin 217
anti-tetanus immunoglobulin 217
anti-varicella zoster immunoglobulin 217
ANUG 19–20
aphthous ulceration 20
arthritis, acute infective 135–7
arthropod vectors 3
aseptic meningitis 9–10
  in HIV infection 150–2
asymptomatic bacteriuria 83–4
athlete's foot 105–7

bacillary dysentery 1, 58–9, 158, 159
Bacillus cereus food poisoning 67–9
bacterial pneumonia 32
bacteriuria, asymptomatic 83–4
BCG 208–10
bilharzia 170–2
biliary tract infections 80–1
black water fever 163
blepharitis 113–14
body fluids, contamination with 2
body lice 2, 101–3
boils 97–9
botulism 67–9
  vaccination 217
bronchiolitis, acute 37–8
bronchitis, chronic, infective
    exacerbations 35–7
bronchopneumonia, infective
    exacerbations 35–7
brucellosis 156, 183, 191–2
'bull neck' 17

Campylobacter spp., gastroenteritis
    associated 57–8
cancrum oris 20
candidiasis
  in HIV infection 144–5
  oral 20–1, 144–5
  vaginal 90–3
carbuncles 97–9
cardiac infections 45–51
cat-scratch fever 193
CDC Group I disease 141
CDC Group II disease 142
CDC Group III disease 142
CDC Group IV disease 142
cellulitis 94–6
  orbital 112–14
central nervous system infection
    5–12
  in HIV infection 150–52
cerebellar ataxia 116
cerebral abscess 5–6
cerebral malaria 163
chalazion 113–14
chancroid 87–9
Charcot's biliary triad 80
chickenpox 115–17
cholangitis, acute 80–1
cholecystitis, acute 80–1
cholera 158, 159
  vaccination 211–12
Clostridium botulinum food poisoning
    67–9
Clostridium perfringens food poisoning
    67–9
CMV infection 183, 186–9
  in HIV infection 144–5
  retinopathy due to 150–2
coeliac disease 158
'cold sores' 19
colitis 63–4
common cold 21–2
Communicable Disease Surveillance
    Centre 4
community, control of infection in 4
condyloma lata 87–9
condylomata acuminata 87–9
congenital rubella syndrome 118, 119
Congo-Crimea virus infection 176–9
conjunctivitis 108–10
consultant in communicable disease
    control 4